D1601670

Women, food
and families

Women, food and families

Nickie Charles *and* Marion Kerr

Manchester University Press
Manchester and New York
Distributed exclusively in the USA and Canada
by **St. Martin's Press** Inc., New York

Published by Manchester University Press
Oxford Road, Manchester M13 9PL, UK
and Room 400, 175 Fifth Avenue, New York, NY 10010, USA

Distributed exclusively in the USA and Canada
by St. Martin's Press, Inc.,
175 Fifth Avenue, New York, NY 10010, USA

British Library cataloguing in publication data

Charles, Nickie
  Women, food and families.
  1. Great Britain. Families. Nutrition.
  Attitudes of women
  I. Title II. Kerr, Marion
  613′.2′088004

Library of Congress cataloging in publication data applied for

ISBN 0–7190–1874–9 hardback

Typeset in Great Britain
by Megaron, Cardiff, Wales

Printed in Great Britain
by Anchor Brendon Ltd., Tiptree, Essex

Contents

Foreword and acknowledgements

The research on which this book is based was carried out by us jointly in the Department of Sociology, University of York. Marion wrote the original research proposal and got the project off the ground, but together we developed ideas and devised detailed questions, and we shared the interviewing and analysis as well as the writing of the research reports. We had intended that the writing of the book would also be equally shared but due to new and competing work commitments this was not possible. If Nickie had not been prepared to take on this task the book might never have become a reality and she has played the major part in producing this account of our findings.

We owe a debt of gratitude to the many people who helped us in the course of our research. Our first thanks must go to all the women who participated in the interviews. It is their experiences on which this book is based and we have learnt a great deal from our discussions with them. For reasons of confidentiality they remain anonymous and, for the same reason, we have changed all the names that appear in the book. Some of them will, perhaps, recognise themselves. All of them gave generously of their time and interest.

Linda Bretherton deserves a special mention for her transcription of hundreds of hours of recorded interviews, for her typing of the research reports and for bearing with us and the project for four and a half years. Diana Estep and Lyn Langford shared the interviewing with us and their approach often added new dimensions to the topics covered during the interviews. Dr Luis Valenzuela painstakingly counted and coded the diary material, Dr Alison Black provided invaluable advice on the interpretation of the diary findings, Dr Rob Fletcher guided us through the complexities of computer analysis and Professor Laurie Taylor gave his support to the research project from its earliest stages. York District Health Authority greatly facilitated our selection of sample families and the research was funded by the Health Education Council. We thank them all.

We also wish to thank Professor Bill Williams of the University College, Swansea, for his support of the book and for the secretarial time that was made available for it to be typed. Carol Cook (and friends) have been responsible for this latter process and our thanks go to them. Needless to say, any shortcomings and omissions in the following pages remain entirely our responsibility.

1

Introduction

This is a book about women and food. And because it is about women and food it is also about men and children and families; very specific families – those which contain pre-school age children; families where children are learning to eat and mothers are trying to teach them the rights and wrongs of mealtime behaviour. It is a book which is written from a sociological perspective: precisely what this is we try to demonstrate below. Food has only recently become interesting to sociologists. In a textbook published in 1981 it was still possible to write: 'Eating habits are simply a matter of fashion and individual taste' (p. 7, Bilton *et al.*, 1981). During the course of this book we hope to demonstrate that nothing could be further from the truth and that eating habits are fundamentally influenced, if not determined, by social factors such as gender, age and class.

Before we discuss the study that we carried out and our methodology we feel it is important to situate our work in its theoretical context. We therefore begin this chapter with a discussion of our theoretical assumptions and then go on to describe our methodology and some of the important social characteristics of the women and their families.

There is now a considerable feminist literature on the ways in which women, within the family, are crucial to the reproduction of the work force on both a daily and generational basis (Barrett, 1980; Burton, 1986; McIntosh, 1984; Wilson, 1977). This reproduction takes place at both the material and ideological levels. For instance, women within the family provide the worker with meals, clean his house, keep him happy and satisfy his sexual 'needs' (Wilson, 1977). Similarly, women satisfy the material needs of children by feeding them, cleaning them, playing with them and loving them. However, there is also an important ideological dimension to this process. Children learn, initially within the family and later at school, which ways of behaving are acceptable. They learn to obey the authority of adults, particularly men; they learn the behaviour appropriate to their gender, and they learn their position in the social division of labour and begin to shape their aspirations accordingly (Barrett, 1980; Delamont, 1980; Oakley, 1982; Sharpe, 1978). This process can be conceptualised as part of the reproduction of ideologies and social divisions which are constitutive of the social order. Bourdieu, among others, has argued that this process of social reproduction takes place constantly in the way we live our daily lives. Practices within the family which are totally taken for granted are, therefore, constantly reproducing social divisions and ideologies (Althusser, 1971; Bourdieu, 1977). The food we eat and the way we eat it can also be approached from this perspective. Food practices can be regarded as one of the ways in which important social relations and divisions are symbolised, reinforced and reproduced on a daily basis. From this theoretical perspective emerges one of our central questions: how do food practices contribute to the reproduction of the social order? More specifically we are asking how social divisions of gender, age and class are reproduced through food practices and how does food relate to the family and patriarchal familial ideology (Barrett, 1980; Murcott, 1982 and 1983).

This concern with food and the way it relates to social divisions and relations of power is not altogether new. Christine Delphy has pointed to the differential consumption of certain status foods within peasant families in France. There meat, which was often in short supply, and alcohol were reserved for men. Women and children ate foods of lesser status and women imposed this denial on themselves through the internalisation of dominant values about the nature of men's as opposed to women's 'needs' (Delphy, 1979). So-called poverty studies in this country at the beginning of the century showed that within the family food consumption was differentiated along lines of age and gender and that women were past mistresses at practising self-denial (Pember Reeves, 1984; Spring Rice, 1981; Rowntree, 1913). Similarly, historical studies and contemporary surveys show that there are strong class patterns in the food and drink that people consume (Boyd-Orr, 1936; NFS, 1984). Sociological studies of child-rearing practices have similarly pointed to class differences in food practices, particularly in the organisation of meals and the behaviour that is expected from children at mealtimes (Newson and Newson, 1970 and 1976; Nicod, 1980). These findings should alert us to the possible differences that may exist between the working-class family and the bourgeois family (Donzelot, 1979). Do food practices within the bourgeois or middle-class family tend to reproduce a more individualised unit than those that exist within working-class families? Is inter-family or even class solidarity differentially affected by the food practices within families from different classes? In this context it is interesting that, historically, changing food habits within the middle classes have eventually influenced food practices within the working class. The consumption of tea is one example as is that of white bread. What were once the preserve of the bourgeoisie are now universally consumed (Boyd-Orr, 1936; Doyal, 1981; Wardle, 1977). Our most tradi-tional food, the potato, was introduced from abroad and first eaten by the aristocracy, but it now seems so much part of our national diet that its foreign ancestry is almost forgotten. M. F. K. Fisher writes of the way potatoes were introduced to Europe – initially for the delight of the upper classes.

In Peru, the Spanish found *papas* growing in the early 1500s, and the monk Hieronymus Cardan took them back with him to his own people. The Italians liked them, and then the Belgians.
    About that time, Sir Walter Raleigh found a potato in the American South, and carried it back to his estate near Cork. Some say it was a yam he had, thought strongly aphrodisiac by the Elizabethans. Some say it was a white potato. A German statute thanks Raleigh for bringing it to Europe. On the other hand, the Spanish claim recogni-tion for its European introduction. (p. 22, Fisher, 1983)

So the pejorative 'foreign food' often uttered by those with conservative tastes in food could also have been applied to their beloved potato, mainstay of family eating in Britain today. The class movement of food habits is interesting and indicates that what the middle classes eat today the working classes eat

tomorrow. It also indicates that the diet differs according to
social class and that the today and tomorrow indicate a
permanent and real divide.

Anthropologists have paid more attention to food than
sociologists (Douglas, 1982; Lévi-Strauss, 1966; Shostak, 1983).
They have long been aware that food carries messages about
social status and the relations between people. Food reflects
and symbolises social relations, it has a part to play in
cementing and reinforcing social relations and can be a
powerful means of inclusion in or exclusion from social groups
(Douglas, 1984). The humble cup of tea offered to a visitor
carries a message of welcome; its absence carries a different
message, one that we all understand.

As food reflects social status it also carries its own social
values. And the values placed on foods are systematised in the
form of food ideologies (Wardle, 1977) which order foods in a
hierarchy (Twigg, 1983) and attach different meanings and
attributes to them. Thus within the dominant food ideology of
western culture meat, particularly red meat, is highly valued
and carries a high social status while vegetables and pulses
occupy a position at the lower end of the hierarchy. Red meat is
associated with strength and virility while other foods are
'weaker' and some, such as horse meat, is too strong to eat at all
(at least within British food culture) (Twigg, 1983; Wardle,
1977). Food ideologies also define what foods are appropriate for
what social occasions; for instance, a roast means Sunday at
home with the family while a multi-coloured cake in the shape of
a train with four candles means that a treasured child has
reached her fourth birthday and is celebrating. Thus food is not
simply nourishment for the body, it is weighted down with
meanings and messages, its use is socially defined (Barthes,
1979).

This is not to say that meanings are static, they can and do
change over time. We have only to think of white bread, once a
status symbol, now a necessary 'filler', tomorrow usurped by the
wholemeal loaf. Barthes is among those who argue that the
meanings attached to food are socially determined. Coffee, once
considered a 'stimulant to the nervous system', is now associated with 'rest and even relaxation. It is that coffee is felt to be
not so much of a substance as a circumstance' (p. 172-3, Barthes,

1979). He argues that all foods, in modern society, are associated with some sort of activity.

Activity, work, sports, effort, leisure, celebration – every one of these situations is expressed through food . . . In the past only festive occasions were signalised by food in any positive and organised manner . . . food is . . . charged with signifying the situation in which it is used. (p. 172, Barthes, 1979)

So food carries meanings and its use and consumption indicate the nature of the social occasion. Its differential consumption by different participants in these social occasions is also a reflection of their status and power. Food therefore carries messages about the nature of the social occasion and about the social relations pertaining between the participants.

Although most anthropological and emergent sociological studies which look at food practices confine their attention to food consumption, and we are proposing to do the same, food production must not be forgotten. Jack Goody has attempted to link food consumption to production in various societies (Goody, 1982), and although we are not proposing to include an analysis of food production in this book we feel it important to emphasise that all we write about is fundamentally influenced by the capitalist nature of food production. Food is *politically* important both here and in the Third World. Here we have so-called diseases of affluence such as obesity and bowel disease; in the Third World people are dying of starvation. Enough food *is* produced to go round, but instead of going to where it is needed it ends up as 'mountains' somewhere in the western world (Tudge, 1979). This global problem stems from the dominance of agribusiness and the production of food for profit (Doyal, 1981; Hayter, 1981). It is part of the historical process of capitalist expansion and affects women as *producers* of food as well as women as consumers. It is the production of food that determines what is available for consumption, and the fact that in capitalist societies food production is geared to profit rather than need is bound to have profound effects on our diet (Wright, 1981). Here, however we take this context as given, it is one of the powerful constraints within which women have to operate in order to feed their families.

There is a third strand to our analysis. In the face of mounting medical evidence there is growing concern about the nature of the western diet, witness the NACNE and COMA reports for instance. The obvious answer to this would be to change the type of food produced; changes in diet would have to follow. But in the absence of the political will to do this, and the example of government inactivity in the face of the cigarette companies shows how difficult it is to get governments to move against big business (Doyal, 1981), it is essential to generate public pressure on food manufacturers to produce more 'healthy' foods. This is, to a certain extent, happening. But in order to change people's food habits, if they are perceived as the problem, it is also necessary to understand why certain foods are eaten rather than others and what cultural pressures produce change. If change is desirable, then it is important to understand the forces which shape and maintain the status quo.

On the one hand foods for individual consumption are determined by production, but on the other hand ideologies, practices and cultural values also influence what is produced and what is available for consumption. This is the level at which our analysis takes place. Production, its capitalist nature and the need to change unhealthy methods of production are taken as given. We concentrate on the other, perhaps superstructural factors which affect why people eat what they do. It could even be argued that food production is a side issue – meat and two veg is the meal that people in families eat, never mind that the meat is full of hormones and the vegetables full of pesticide residues. Changing the methods of food production will solve these problems, and change *does* seem to be taking place at this level. But what is it that leads us to eat food put together in the form of a meal consisting of meat and two veg? Why is it so resistant to change even when we *know* it is probably not doing us any good? These are the practical issues that we wish to explore.

Centrally, however, the book is concerned with women. Within the family woman's place is defined as being in the kitchen, cooking for men and children, feeding them, nourishing them. It is women whose lives revolve around food and they will form the focus of our book.

Again, a concern with women and food is not new to feminists. Witness the books written on women's problematic relationship to food, women's eating disorders, women's relationship to their mothers and daughters (Chernin, 1983 and 1986; Lawrence, 1984; MacLeod, 1981; Orbach, 1981). These feminists, however, all write from the perspective of women's psychology. Our analysis, as we said at the outset, is sociological and as such it focuses on the social factors which shape women's experiences as the servers and providers of food within families.

Methodology

Two hundred women with at least one child who was under school age were each interviewed twice during 1982 and 1983. The interviews were separated by a gap of a fortnight, during which time the women kept diary records of the food and drink consumed by everyone in their household. As our study was sociological rather than nutritional, we did not ask that the women weigh and measure what they ate, but they did give some indication of the relative size of helpings eaten by different family members. This enabled us, in the second interview, to ask about the different amounts of food eaten by men and women, adults and children, as well as discussing other aspects of the family's diets. The interviews were tape-recorded and, later, transcribed and coded for the computer. The material we have is therefore qualitative, as we included many open-ended questions which gave the women the chance to talk freely, and quantitative, as the sample was large enough to produce useful statistical data.

The interviews covered a very wide range of topics all of which involved food within the family. We asked women about the allocation of tasks such as food shopping, preparation and cooking and decision making. We explored the factors which led to certain foods being eaten rather than others, such as partners' and children's likes and dislikes, the cost of food, its nutritional values, and so on. The role of food within marriage and the way that giving up work and having children affects the food eaten were talked about, as was the way that men influence the family's diet. We asked women about the daily diet and how it changed at weekends and on holidays, and we asked them to describe the sorts of food and drink they consumed on special occasions such as Christmas and birthdays. We talked to them in some detail about feeding children, about the relationship between food and health and about their experiences of dieting. And we also explored the influence of kin, health care professionals and the media on the way women fed their families. As we will see below, the assumption we made to begin with – that women are generally the ones who are responsible for feeding themselves, their partners and their children – was completely justified. This assumption led us to interview women on this topic rather than men and in only one household did we find that cooking and food preparation were largely carried out by the woman's partner. The interviews, therefore, covered almost all aspects of feeding a family and some of them lasted several hours. A discussion of food, we found, although seemingly a 'safe' topic, often turned out to be the key to unlocking all sorts of problematic areas of women's lives. This was particularly true of that part of the interview where we asked the women whether they had ever dieted. This question often revealed all sorts of anxieties and tensions surrounding food and eating which had not become apparent before.

The focus of the research was initially on the formation of eating habits in young children. But our interests were wider than this. We felt that children learn to eat within a specific social context, the family, and they not only learn to differentiate between what is appropriate to eat and what is not (cat food or sand may be just as appetising to a small child as shepherd's pie) and the order and combination in which food is eaten, they also learn about social divisions of gender and age. We therefore thought it important to explore these divisions insofar as they are involved in the presentation of food to children.

The women were selected for interview in a specific geographical area in the north of England. We do not think that this means our findings are geographically specific, particularly in the light of Ann Murcott's work in South Wales and the findings of Mack and Lansley for their book *Poor Britain* (Mack and Lansley, 1985; Murcott, 1982). However, ethnic minorities were virtually unrepresented amongst our sample. This reflects the demographic composition of the area in which the research was carried out and means that our findings are specific to white British households.

The major focus of our research was on the reproduction of divisions of gender, age and class through food practices.

Women's relationship to food forms the main focus of the discussion which follows, but we are also centrally concerned with the ways in which class divisions are represented and reinforced through food practices and the way class mediates women's experiences as providers of food within the family. Given the problematic nature of definitions of social class and the even more problematic nature of the relation between gender divisions and class, we felt that we could not simply classify the women and their families according to the occupation of their partners. We felt that this classification would obscure the attitudes and values that shape practices within the family and that, for women at least, may come from their family background, their education and their own occupation and experience in the job market. For these reasons we decided to classify women according to their own current or last full-time occupation. Men, even unemployed men, we classified similarly. We used the Registrar General's classification of occupations so as to maintain comparability with other studies.

The test of our methodology lies in its explanatory value, and, as we show in the pages that follow, women's social class seems to have greater impact on many aspects of family eating habits and patterns than does that of men. We have in fact used both women's and men's occupational class, usually selecting for presentation the one which shows the clearest correlation.

The women and their families

Almost all (181) the women we spoke to were married and living with the father of their children; a further seven were cohabiting, ten were lone parents and two became lone parents between the first and second interviews. Most (154) of the women had one or two children although there were a few (10) families with four or more children.

In 8 of the families there were step-children present. Three of the women who were lone parents still lived at home with their parent/s, but all the others had set up separate households. Only two of these households included people who were not part of the immediate nuclear family; in one the woman's semi-invalid father-in-law was present and a friend lived with another family. Thus most of the women were living in a household containing their own nuclear family, the so-called average family of husband, wife and one or two children. Of the households, 105 contained pre-school age children only, although in 76 children of pre-school and school age were present, in 7 the children's ages ranged from pre-school through to 16 and over, in 8 all the children were at school and in 4 there were either pre-school age children or school age children *and* children of 16 and over.

Most women (159) lived in homes they and their partners owned or were buying with a mortgage, 34 lived in rented accommodation and three were living with their parent/s. A further 4 either were living in tied accommodation or were in the process of buying a council house. Most of the women (146) lived near to their parents or parents-in-law with only a quarter of them not having either set of parents relatively nearby. This seemed to be linked to social class: 55% of families where the male partner was in social class I/II did not live near either set of parents, while 57% of families in social class IV/V lived near both sets of parents.

The ages of the women ranged fairly widely. The majority (154) were between 20 and 34, 27 were between 35 and 39, and 9 were over 40. Most of them (148) had left school at 15 or 16 (the minimum school leaving age) with 24 having stayed at school until they were 18 and 28 going on to further or higher education. Almost without exception the women had worked full-time before having children and the nature of their jobs is shown in Table 1.1. Most women's work had been concentrated in the service sectors, particularly secretarial and clerical work, and women in the professions worked exclusively in the areas of health, education and the social services. However, at the time of interview, unsurprisingly given the fact that they had children under school age, 119 (59.5%) of them were not involved in paid employment outside the home. Those who were, were mainly working part-time so that they could combine their child-care responsibilities with paid work. Usually this meant that they worked an evening 'twilight' shift which meant that their partners could look after the children while they were out at work.

Other women worked weekends or even nights for similar reasons; this latter pattern was mostly to be found amongst nurses. The few women working full-time were able to afford

Table 1.1 *Women's last occupation before having children (n = 200) –
no. (%)*

Non-manual skilled:		
Secretarial, clerical	84	(42·0)
Manual unskilled:		
Process workers, cleaners, waitresses	30	(15·0)
Manual skilled:		
Cooks, care assistants	10	(5·0)
Non-manual unskilled:		
Shop assistants	20	(10·0)
Health and childcare workers	26	(13·0)
Academic and related professions,		
teachers, social workers	19	(9·5)
Managerial	1	(0·5)
Other:		
Self-employed, worked for partner	3	(1·5)
Never worked	4	(2·0)

help such as nannies or child-minders with their children: they
were usually women from the higher (and better paid) occupational classes. Those women who were working in paid employment worked as process workers and cleaners (22), shop
assistants (16), secretaries and clerical workers (4); one was a
cook and 17 were teachers or nurses. Six of the women worked
for their partners, typing up bills or doing the accounts, and 6
ran catalogues or were involved in freelance work of one sort or
another. A further 2 were students and 5 were on maternity
leave. This spread of occupations is typical of women's employment: they are generally to be found in low status and low
paid sectors of the work force, particularly after they have had
children. This is probably because most women have to take up
jobs with hours of work that fit in with their child-care
responsibilities (Charles and Brown, 1981) and these are mainly
to be found in the service sector, such as shops and restaurants,
where part-time work abounds, and in factories where twilight
shifts are organised with precisely this sector of the labour force
in mind. Men's jobs, on the other hand, are not circumscribed in
this way and the jobs that the men living with the women we
interviewed held were spread across a wide range of occupations. Over a third of the men (39%) were working in skilled,
manual work such as drivers or skilled tradesmen and a number

of them were self-employed; 20% of the men were in professional
occupations, such as teachers, architects, solicitors and doc-
tors. This can be seen in Table 1.2.

Table 1.2   *Partner's present occupation (n = 200) – no. (%)*

Skilled manual	57	(29)
Other manual	19	(10)
Self-employed		
(primarily skilled manual)	22	(11)
Non-manual	30	(15)
Professional	39	(20)
Managerial	13	(7)
Unemployed	6	(3)
Others: student, in prison	4	(2)
No partner	10	(5)

From this it can be seen that six of the men were unemployed
at the time of interview. Without exception they had all
previously been in manual occupations. One of the men whose
occupation was professional was not in paid employment when
we interviewed his partner. However, he was not claiming
supplementary or unemployment benefit and was working on
some research. As he did not regard himself as unemployed we
have not counted him among the unemployed men.

A majority of the women we interviewed came from occupational class IIIN, as defined by their present or last full-time
occupation, while the men were not concentrated in any
particular sector of the occupational hierarchy.[1] This reflects
the way women's jobs are concentrated in particular areas of
'white collar' work such as secretarial and clerical occupations.
These figures are shown in Table 1.3.

Women were most likely to have married men from their own
occupational class with the exception of women in secretarial
or clerical jobs (IIIN). They were more likely to have married
men in skilled manual occupations (IIIM). This is shown in
Table 1.4.

As would be expected, the earnings of the women and their
partners varied considerably, ranging from those who were
dependent on supplementary benefit, which during 1981/82 was

Table 1.3 *Social class distribution of women and men – no. (%).*
Occupational class of women and men is defined according to their own
current or last full-time occupation

	Women		Men	
I/II	42	(21·0)	60	(31·6)
IIIN	104	(52·0)	28	(14·7)
IIIM	29	(14·5)	78	(41·1)
IV/V	18	(9·0)	21	(11·1)
Student/not given	7	(3·5)	3	(1·6)
Total	200	(100·0)	190	(100·0)

Table 1.4 *Extent of marriage outside own class – no. (%)*

Women's occupational class:	I/II		IIIN		IIIM		IV/V		Other/not given		Total	
I/II	27	(64)	26	(25)	6	(21)	1	(6)			60	(30·0)
IIIN	4	(10)	17	(16)	3	(10)	3	(17)	1	(14·3)	28	(14·0)
IIIM	6	(14)	51	(49)	11	(38)	5	(28)	5	(71·4)	78	(39·0)
IV/V	3	(7)	6	(6)	6	(21)	6	(33)			21	(10·5)
Single parent	1	(2)	3	(3)	3	(10)	3	(17)			10	(5·0)
Other/not given	1	(2)	1	(1)	0	·	0		1	(14·3)	3	(1·5)
Total	42	(100)	104	(100)	29	(100)	18	(100)	7	(100·0)	200	(100·0)

£23.25 for a single person, £37.75 for a couple and £7.90 for each
child under 11, to those who were earning joint salaries of
around £20,000 per year. We classified the families into low
income households (20), low/middle income households (56),
middle income households (58) and high income households (11).
Low income households had a man bringing in less than £80 per
week; low/middle income families were characterised by a male
take home wage of £80–£100 per week; in middle income
households men earned more than £100 per week but less than
£10,000 per year; households where men earned over this
amount were classified as high income. These categories are
relative to our sample. Average gross earnings during 1982 were
£150.50 per week. This classification relates to men's income
only, for though around a third of the women worked outside the
home and their earnings were significant in terms of the family

budget they did not affect households' placings in terms of their broad income band. In addition to this, 17 households were in receipt of social security benefits and 27 of the women did not know what their partners were earning. If the poverty line is taken to be the supplementary benefit level and the crude assumption is made that households consisted of two adults and two children under 11, then 37 of the families were living at a level which was fairly near this line.

The families who are included in the analysis of actual food consumption over the two week period during which the women kept a diary of the food and drink consumed show a similar class distribution to the main sample. This is shown in Table 1.5.

Table 1.5 *Social class composition of main sample (n = 200) and sub-sample (n = 157) based on women's current or last full-time occupation – no. (%)*

	Main sample		Sub-sample	
I/II	42	(21)	34	(22)
IIIN	104	(52)	81	(52)
IIIM	29	(15)	22	(14)
IV/V	18	(9)	14	(10)
Student/not given	7	(4)	6	(4)

Although our initial sampling method was designed to ensure that every household included at least one pre-school age child, and we stratified the sample according to the age of the pre-school age child, children of other ages were inevitably included. Their food and drink consumption was recorded by the women and so when we analyse these data we include all children under the age of 12 years. Their distribution by the woman's social class is shown in Table 1.6.

As can be seen, by far the highest proportion of children is in the under 5 age group; this is true for every social class and reflects our initial sampling method. Clearly our findings for this age group and for adults are likely to be the most reliable, but we feel that patterns among the older children are interesting enough to be included, although we must bear in mind that the sample on which they are based is relatively small. The over 11 age group, however, is problematic and is not included in our

Table 1.6   *Age distribution of children by social class of woman – no. (%)*

	I/II	IIIN	IIIM	IV/V	Student/ not given	Total
Under 5 years old	55 (80)	120 (76)	33 (77)	18 (64)	11 (73)	237 (76·0)
5–11 years	10 (14)	25 (16)	10 (23)	5 (18)	2 (13)	52 (16·6)
12 years and over	4 (6)	12 (8)	—	5 (18)	2 (13)	23 (7·4)
Total	69 (100)	157 (100)	43 (100)	28 (100)	15 (100)	312 (100·0)

analysis of the diary material. It was a highly diverse group and included some children who were at work while others were at school. They tended to eat away from home much more frequently than other family members and by no means always participated in the main family meal. In consequence, their diary records are frequently inadequate and we have, with regret, taken the decision to exclude them from our analysis. For the purposes of exploring differences in consumption between adults and children within families we have, therefore, focused on the consumption patterns of children under the age of 12.

Our analysis of actual consumption is based on the two-week diary records of 157 of our 200 families. Most women were very conscientious in their diary-keeping and only 5 did not fill in the diaries they were given; a further 12 women provided an inadequate diary record. The remaining families were excluded from our analysis here because during the period of diary-keeping their pattern of eating had been disrupted through illness (15), holidays (5) or partner's absence from the home (4). In addition 2 women experienced marital separation during the course of the study. Not surprisingly, this disrupted their diary-keeping although both of them decided they wished to continue with the interviews.

The sub-sample for whom we have accurate diary records of everyday family eating comprises 151 two-parent families and 6 single parent families, including a total of 312 children. The male partner was unemployed in 6 families.

These then are the women and their families. In the following pages we explore the place of food and eating habits within the family and the ways in which they relate to social divisions of gender, age and class. Our discussion falls roughly into three parts. Firstly, we explore the relation between food and the family in both its nuclear and extended form. We concentrate specifically on the way food practices contribute to the reproduction of familial ideology and patriarchal power relations. We then go on to look at food practices within the family. We explore the implications of the gender division of labour which characterised our families and food practices resulting from it for women's relation to men, children, their own sexuality and health. In the third part we turn our attention to the situation of families within the wider society and look at the effect of a stratified class system on the foods we eat. Finally, we draw together our major findings, discussing some of the theoretical and policy implications of our research.

Note

1   Women's and men's occupations were grouped according to the Registrar General's classification of occupations. Thus professional and managerial occupations are grouped in occupational class I; semi-professional occupations such as teaching and nursing, in occupational class II; other non-manual occupations, such as clerical and secretarial work, in occupational class IIIN; occupational class IIIM comprises skilled manual work, occupational class IV semi-skilled manual work and occupational class V, unskilled manual work.

2

Proper meals: proper families

Food is a central part of many family occasions, ranging from those that take place so often that we totally take them for granted to those that are annual or even less frequent events and as such are special and memorable. In the former category are the daily main meal and Sunday 'dinner' and in the latter category such events as Christmas, birthdays, weddings and christenings. In this chapter we will explore the food and drink that people consume together as a family, concentrating particularly on 'Christmas dinner', 'Sunday dinner', and the daily 'proper meal' or 'cooked dinner'. We will argue that food is important to the social reproduction of the family in both its nuclear and extended forms, and that food practices help to maintain and reinforce a coherent ideology of the family throughout the social structure. Meals can be seen as symbolising the important social relations of power and subordination that exist within the family. They function as a means of maintaining and reproducing a specific aspect of the social order, the family and the age and gender divisions which characterise it. Here we will concentrate on those aspects of family food practices which unite families across classes; in later chapters we will explore those aspects which divide families from one another in terms of status and occupational grouping.

Food is important to family ideology. In terms of this ideology, an important aspect of women's role within the family is to provide proper family meals for men and children. The woman-wife-mother prepares and cooks food that is 'wholesome' and 'nutritious', the epitome of 'good, home-cooking'. The

most important meal she cooks in the day is the main meal
which ideally should be eaten by the family *as a family*; i.e., they
should eat it together sitting round a table, talking to each other
and enjoying the food and each other's company. This is seen as
an important part of family life and something for which women
are responsible. Similarly, the Sunday dinner of roast meat,
vegetables and potatoes is another important family meal.
Indeed, Sunday seems to be defined as a day for the family, for
visiting relatives if they live near enough, and for sharing food
with them in the form of Sunday dinner or tea. Christmas, and
the food associated with it, is also defined as a time of year when
families, some of whose members may be scattered far and wide,
come together and share food with each other. These three types
of meals, the proper meal of daily family eating, the Sunday
roast with potatoes and vegetables and the Christmas dinner,
are part and parcel of the ideology of the family. They are
regarded as a central part of family life and, indeed, the
production and consumption of these meals in some way define
a family *as* a family. In terms of this ideology families are the
same throughout the social structure, they have the same
values, share the same beliefs and eat the same food in the same
form. In this sense, food practices are important to the reproduction of the family and to the reproduction of family ideology.
The shared experience of family meals, such as Sunday dinner,
unites families ideologically and culturally across other social
divisions such as those of class. Of course, food practices *also*
reproduce divisions, precisely those of class and ethnicity, but
in this chapter we wish to concentrate on those aspects of family
food practices which tend to unify across society.

Let us turn our attention first to the more mundane and
taken-for-granted aspects of family eating, the daily 'proper'
meal and the Sunday 'dinner'. We begin with a discussion of the
nature of the proper meal as it is so crucial to the argument we
present in the rest of the book.

The proper meal

For the majority of the women a proper meal was clearly taken
to be a meal made up of meat (sometimes fish), potatoes and
vegetables. The other meals of the day were given different

names – lunch, breakfast or tea – and these also had character-istic properties, but the term 'proper meal' was never used to refer to any but the main meal of the day, the cooked dinner. The Sunday dinner, with a similar content but in the more elaborate form of the roast, was the proper meal *par excellence*. The regular provision of such meals was the ideal towards which women were striving.

The proper meal of meat and two vegetables was often defined in opposition to a 'snack' or 'snack-type' meal which usually constituted the non-main meal of the day. A snack was bread based and perhaps included a sweet element; it was also often defined as not being cooked. This was sometimes even the case if the meal being discussed consisted of something like poached egg on toast. Indeed, whether or not food preparation is defined as cooking seems to depend on the end product of the process. If the product is a proper meal then it has been cooked, whereas heating food up, making toast or boiling an egg is not classed as cooking. Thus, lunch and tea, when they are non-main meals, may be 'prepared' but they are unlikely to be cooked. On the other hand, we are all familiar with a 'cooked breakfast' consisting of bacon, eggs and so on, which is this meal in its most proper form.

As the proper meal is structurally linked to the Sunday dinner so is a snack related to the traditional Sunday tea, the 'proper tea' as it was referred to by several of the women. This type of tea, the non-main meal on a Sunday, is based on bread with sweet elements, such as fruit, biscuits, cake or pudding, and perhaps a salad. However, a 'snack' often included only one or two of the elements appropriate to a 'proper tea' and this meant that its status as a meal was ambiguous. It is in this context that we can also understand the reason why, for many of the women and more of the men, a salad was not considered to be a 'proper meal'. It is part of the 'proper tea' rather than being part of a proper meal of meat and two vegetables. However, if a salad is served with meat and potatoes – rather than bread – its status can be elevated to that of a 'proper meal'. Fruit is also traditionally an element of 'proper tea'. The inclusion of fresh fruit and salad in the 'proper tea' perhaps helps to explain why they were not often eaten as part of the main meal.

The midday meal rather than tea was the non-main meal of the day in most households on weekdays and reflected the structure of the traditional 'proper tea' based on bread. However, it was clearly regarded as a snack or a 'snack-type' meal by most of the women and occupied a less important place than the 'proper meal'. It is interesting to note that breakfast was never referred to as a snack no matter what it consisted of.

We should also mention that there seem to be definite rules about the order in which elements of meals are eaten. It is not only the main meal that this is applied to. Lunch and even children's birthday teas are structured inasmuch as the savoury course is eaten before the sweet course.

Meals, particularly proper meals, are viewed by the women as an important part of family life and, as such, are not only defined by their content. In contrast to a 'snack' a proper meal is often seen as a social occasion; a chance for all the family to sit down and eat a meal together:

A proper meal is an occasion, for want of a better word, where everybody will sit down together and take time over eating a meal and do it properly, whereas a snack is something that you could just eat while you were doing something else and on your own, whereas a meal is, I think, an occasion.

It also takes place in a specific social context:

A proper meal is when you sit down with a knife and fork and there's potatoes and meat and veg and whatever. That's what I call the main meal like when I do the meal for when John comes in and we all sit down for . . . it's the main meal of the day that. It's the one that I put more thought into because we all sit down to eat this meal.

All the family eat a proper meal sitting down together and it is cooked by the woman with more attention than is given to the other meals of the day. For most of our families eating a proper meal also involved eating at table: 'Well I like Sunday lunch, I enjoy it. It's really the only time that we all sit down together and talk, you know, sitting round the table.' The proper meal, therefore, whether it takes the form of the Sunday joint or the more ordinary weekday meat and two vegetables, is seen as an occasion for all the family to be together. Indeed, the presence of all family members is required for a proper meal to be provided. The proper meal is regarded in a fundamental way as a family meal and is itself constitutive of the family as a cohesive social unit. One of the women we spoke to expressed this clearly when asked whether she thought it important for a woman to be able to cook:

Very important, it's part of the family existence, it's one of the main occasions in the day when everybody gets together to eat and chat and if you've got rubbish in front of you you're miserable, aren't you? I think men enjoy it, most of them do. If you put beans on toast down in front of them every day they'd soon go off it.

This indicates the importance of a proper meal eaten together as a family in keeping the family together as a social entity and the woman's key role in the cooking of such a meal. Many of the women expressed similar views:

I think they are very, very important because I think it's the time when the family come together, and it's really the only time they come together as a family. Which is why we all sit down and have a chance to talk. I think it's the most important part of the day apart from cooking.

In most households mealtimes are not only about eating, they are a time to be together as a family and to talk to each other. In fact, 127 (63·5%) of the women said that they thought it was important to talk at mealtimes while only 38 (19%) said it was not important.

Table manners were also felt to be important to a family meal. Most of the women felt that it was important for a child to learn table manners in order to be able to take them out and not be embarrassed by them; in other words, so that their behaviour at mealtimes was socially acceptable. One woman expressed this clearly. She was asked why she thought table manners important and said: 'For the comfort of other people. Especially if you go out. It's pretty awful taking a messy child out to a restaurant.'

Thus a proper meal is defined not only by its contents but by the way it is eaten and what happens during the meal in terms of behaviour. It is also defined by who is present. It is ideally a meal which is a 'family' meal and this, by definition, requires all members of the family to be present. It is also a meal which is cooked by the woman in the household for herself, her partner and her children. Thus if her partner is away at the time of the main meal when a 'proper' family meal is normally cooked and eaten it has an effect on the content of the meal. Of the women's partners, 132 had been absent from the main meal at some time or another and 47% of these women ate differently when their partners were away, 31% ate at a different time and 14% ate in a different place.

The content usually changed from those elements appropriate to a proper meal to elements more appropriate – in the women's own views – to a 'snack-type' meal: 'If Greg's been away I've not bothered to cook proper meals – proper meals in as much as a cooked meal. I probably wouldn't go to the trouble of cooking myself meat, vegetables and potatoes.' The content could also be influenced by children's preferences in ways which were not usually possible when their fathers were present. Such changes begin to reveal the complex power relations which structure the provision of the proper meal. One woman, for example, told us about the type of meal she and the children ate in the absence of her partner: 'If he's away then it's usually on toast, anything on toast.' Her son, Robert, prefers this type of meal to a proper meal:

Robert he does like sandwiches but if he's taken one to school he'll often come home and say, 'Is it a butty for tea?' and if I say, 'No, it's a cooked meal,' he'll say 'Ugh!' He'd rather sit down to one [sandwich] so if I've got an excuse not to cook then I won't.

This excuse arises for her if her partner's away and then the children can choose:

Sometimes when Bob's not here – well I nearly always do when Bob's not here, I say, 'What do you want Robert?' and he'll usually say a sandwich or a boiled egg. So he does get a choice. He gets the choice quite a lot really. The only thing he doesn't get a choice about is the main meal that I've cooked.

Clearly she only cooks a 'proper' main meal if her partner is present, otherwise the main meal becomes a 'snack-type' meal at which the children can choose. The main meal is thus a means of instilling into children the authority of the father in the household: their eating habits have to conform to what is appropriate to him as head of the household. In his (temporary) absence these rules are relaxed and the food conforms to the children's preferences. His presence is therefore necessary for the family to be constituted as a 'proper' family – symbolically represented in the provision of the proper meal.

It was also often considered too much of an effort to cook only for the children when they may not eat a proper meal anyway. The presence of their partner justified the effort expended in a way that children did not. One woman said: 'I can't be bothered to cook if there's just the three of us, Bob inspires me to cook I suppose.'

It was clearly not worth women cooking a proper meal unless the man-husband-father was going to be present to consume it with the rest of the family. It is a family meal which needs the presence of the whole family to justify its preparation.

The presence of children was also considered a necessary condition for the provision of 'proper' meals and several of the women said that they only started cooking 'properly' after the children were born:

> . . . it wasn't really till we had Robert . . . that I had to really get down and think, 'Oh God I've got to do all them blasted meals a day . . . for him', but it was then that I got into it a lot more. It seemed more like a home to me and having it planned that you were going to have a meal and that . . . although we only had one meal a day – but it's nice to have it. You have to make the effort with them [children] yes. I know that if one day, if for some reason we have to have something on toast or something like that I know the next day, well I *feel* the next day I've got to make up for it and do a meal.

It was also seen as necessary for a *woman* to have cooked a meal for it to be considered a *proper* meal. Very often when men were left to provide food for the children they did not produce a proper meal but something that was easier to prepare and did not even involve 'cooking'. Thus a proper meal is also defined by the social relationships within which it is prepared, cooked and eaten. It has to be eaten by all the family members, father, mother and children, and the absence of any of them makes it less likely that a proper meal will be provided. The provision of proper meals is also viewed as an important aspect of the woman's role in the home. One woman, when asked if she thought it was important for a woman to be able to cook, replied:

> Well *I* think it *is*, when they're married, I mean whatever you do when you're single it's up to you, it doesn't matter, but I think you've got

more responsibilities to your children and to your husband and I think you ought to be able to . . .

This was a view shared by most of the women and points to the fact that cooking is seen as a vital part of a woman's domestic responsibilities once she is married. Thus there is a clear sexual division of labour operating in the realm of family food provision which was seen, by many of the women, as fundamental to family life.

The preparation and consumption of 'proper' meals, therefore, represents and reinforces the social divisions of labour and particularly power relations within the family. The dominance of the father is recreated daily through the preparation of a proper meal which is usually eaten by all members of the family together and in which the children have very little if any choice. Meals when the father is absent are different: choice can be exercised and they are not structured in the same way as a proper meal. The wife-mother's own choice is subordinated, first to her partner and then to her children in the provision of meals – whether they are proper meals or not – and, as will become increasingly clear in succeeding chapters, the preparation and cooking of proper meals are seen as vital both to family life in general and to the role of the woman in the household in particular.

Sunday dinner

'Sunday dinner', the proper meal *par excellence*, was eaten regularly by the majority of our families. It was, like the everyday proper meal, often not provided until the arrival of children, and their ability to share a proper meal finally constituted the household unit as a 'proper' family. This 'properness' was then symbolically recreated on a daily and weekly basis with proper meals and Sunday dinner:

Since Alison was 3½ we started having proper Sunday lunches which is something we'd never done before. Before we had children we used to spend most of Sunday in bed anyway, but now we have Sunday lunches and we've even got to the stage when I'm told to put a tablecloth on by Alison and we lay the table and put wine glasses out even if we're not having wine – that kind of thing – so it's a great performance.

In fact, the Sunday dinner was much *more* likely to be eaten together by all family members than were proper meals during the week. This was particularly the case if men worked away from home or arrived home late on weekday evenings. Only 27 out of the 200 women we spoke to did not prepare and eat 'Sunday dinner', and in only 38 families was the main meal on Sunday not eaten together by all family members. In comparison, during the week 76 of the families did not eat their main meal together and on a Saturday 56 did not. Thus for most families the 'Sunday dinner' was eaten by all the family together, and for a substantial number it was eaten as an extended family, either at their own house or that of the women's parents or parents-in-law. Women on low incomes still made every effort to provide their families with a 'Sunday dinner' as well as regular proper meals, but sometimes the only way of doing this was by relying on parents or parents-in-law: 'Every Sunday we go up to my Mam's for our dinner. If I had to get a joint on a weekend I really would be completely out of money.'

It was evident that regular consumption of proper meals and a 'proper' Sunday dinner, whatever the level of income or occupational status of a family, were regarded as an important part of family life. And families that did not eat in this way, whether by choice or necessity, were regarded in some fundamental way as not constituting 'proper' families, and not having a 'proper' family life. It is in this sense that we are arguing that the proper meal and the practices surrounding its provision and consumption are important to the reproduction of the family, characterised as it is by unequal relations of power, and that the proper meal – whether in its weekday, Sunday or Christmas form – is an important component of familial ideology. In practice it brings together the family, it symbolises its existence, and it reproduces the social divisions of age and gender which characterise it.

Thus far we have concentrated on the significance of the daily and weekly forms of the proper meal eaten by the families in our sample. Let us now turn our attention to Christmas, arguably the high point of family eating in the year, and birthdays, which are also important occasions in the life of families with young children.

Christmas dinner

Christmas dinner is the prototype of the proper family meal and
the food involved in the Christmas ritual is fundamentally a
celebration of the coming together of family members. The food
is special and festive and Christmas is a time of indulgence in
foods which are rich (containing ingredients of high status)
and/or are themselves of high status. These foods are usually
roast turkey, Christmas pudding, made with alcohol and eaten
with alcohol sauce, and/or a Christmas cake which, similarly,
contains alcohol. Commonly wine and other alcoholic drinks
are consumed at this time of the year more than at any other.
There is plenty of food and drink for everyone and the normal
restraints on eating and drinking are temporarily lifted; self-
indulgence rather than self-denial is the order of the day.

Christmas dinner itself is marked by status foods, extra
vegetables, different kinds of potatoes, stuffings, sauces, and
often more than one kind of meat. For instance, the turkey can
be stuffed with sausage meat and bacon and sausages are
cooked with it. As well as the main course, many families eat a
starter and, of course, the Christmas pudding, bathed in and
containing alcohol. All this is washed down by alcohol of one
sort or another, even if families never normally drink alcohol at
home during the rest of the year.

The meal that is eaten to celebrate the family at Christmas
time is very similar across the social spectrum; 143 (71·5%) of
our families ate roast turkey and 148 (74%) ate Christmas
pudding. If families did not eat a turkey they ate other meats
that were roasted and were in some way special. The only
exception to this was provided by the four vegetarian families
we spoke to, but their Christmas meals were also special and
festive. Overall, though, 176 (88%) of the families ate a
Christmas meal which consisted, at least partly, of food which
has come to be known as traditional Christmas fare.

Many of the women described their Christmas meal, com-
menting on its structural similarity to normal Sunday dinners
and the over-indulgence that is involved at this time of year:

We generally have a turkey because it's economic, although it lasts too
long, and the trimmings and potatoes, carrots, peas, sprouts and one
other vegetable, mashed potatoes and roast, stuffing and sausages,

bread sauce and cranberry sauce, Christmas pudding and rum sauce. I think you tend to eat a lot more for your Christmas dinner than for other meals and, of course, you have pudding as well, you make pigs of yourselves. We always say, every year, 'Never again, we're not going to have as much next year', but we always do. If you can't enjoy yourself at Christmas when can you do it?

For low income families it was often difficult to buy in extra food at Christmas, and this could mean that they saved money for it all year. One woman described how she managed to make sure Christmas was special even though she did not have very much money:

We pay so much for a hamper every year – we get that off the milkman. We got a meat pack last year didn't we? We paid so much a week, and we got £25 worth, and we got these vouchers and we went to Dewhursts in town. We got everything, it was lovely to have meat you know. We even got steak, so you can tell it was a treat, a real treat – the kids loved it, "Cor, look at what me mam's got in the freezer' – things they'd never seen before.

This pattern of saving for a special meal, usually the ritual Sunday roast, was common among low income families throughout the year: they scrimped on food throughout the week so as to ensure that they could enjoy the traditional Sunday dinner. The process of saving up for Christmas dinner is merely the weekly procedure writ large, and it indicates that despite the exigencies of income, women make a huge effort to provide their families with a special Christmas meal. It is felt to be an important family occasion, and the food appropriate to such an occasion must be provided by hook or by crook.

Christmas Day, a holiday for men and children, is a day of hard work and organising for women. Most of the women we spoke to were the ones who prepared and cooked this meal. In 15 of the families the women's partners helped, and in 7 the men actually cooked the meal. But generally the cooking of this family meal is seen as a woman's task, and is either undertaken by the woman herself in her role as wife and mother or by her and other female relatives. Indeed, some women particularly enjoyed cooking Christmas dinner precisely because 'it is festive and out of the ordinary', and very much resented their husband's attempts to take over the cooking of this particular meal: 'We used to argue about who cooked Christmas dinner because we both wanted to do it. But I always do now. He helps though and makes sauces.' Although women cooked, men might wash up. As one woman commented: 'That is a rule in our family, the ladies do the meal and the men wash up.' However, in most families it was women who cooked Christmas dinner *and* washed up. And although in a few cases men might argue over who was to cook Christmas dinner, *no* women reported arguments over who should prepare and cook the daily round of proper family meals.

Christmas dinner was important as a means of uniting family members who did not normally come together to share food. It is because of this that it has a symbolic significance. It represents the coming together of the extended family and is a means of uniting and reinforcing bonds between family members who may not eat together at any other time of year. In fact, 116 (58%) of our families ate Christmas dinner as an extended family while 71 (35·5%) ate it as a nuclear family. The figure for those eating this meal as an extended family is therefore considerably higher than the number of families celebrating Christmas as a nuclear family.

This points to an extremely significant ideological function of Christmas dinner which distinguishes it from a normal Sunday dinner, and that is that it brings together and, therefore, reinforces the extended family, while the Sunday dinner, together with the proper family meal, reinforces the nuclear family. For most of the women, then, Christmas is essentially an extended family occasion and this can mean that the logistics of the event become fairly complicated:

Since we've got married we've never had a Christmas dinner at home. [Do you take it in turns where to go?] We usually do, yes. I think the first Christmas we had it at my mum's, the second Christmas at my husband's mother's and then we went back to my mum's the third Christmas and the fourth Christmas we had it at my sister's . . . So it is difficult choosing where to go because I suppose each one of us wants to be with our family as well but we've just sort of come to an arrangement where we take it in turns . . . In fact this year I said I wouldn't mind staying at home but I don't know, Christmas dinner for the three of us wouldn't seem the same. My husband comes from a big family – four brothers and four sisters – Christmas dinner there is always nice, there's always lots of people there, it's nice. At my mum's there's always plenty of people there – I can't visualise it on our own.

The turkey, a large bird, is ideally consumed by large numbers of people, otherwise it lasts for too long. One of the women commented on this:

It does tend to depend where we are I suppose but it's just traditional usually. But if Mark and I were left to ourselves at home and we didn't have to bother with anybody else I'd probably do – I'd buy a piece of pork or something different, we wouldn't bother buying turkey for ourselves, in fact we never really have. I did one year and it just sort of sat there for days and days and we got fed up of it. I got too big a one I suppose really. With his parents being here and my parents being at home, there's nobody else for his parents to go to, so either they are with us or we're with them so that really does necessitate turkey, you know, we do the full thing.

It is not only Christmas dinner that is special and shared with the extended family although it is frequently the high spot of the culinary festivities. Many families have a Christmas tea with Christmas cake as well, and others may have more than one Christmas dinner to fit in meals with all the family at some time during the Christmas period: 'We usually go to Dave's mum and dad for Christmas lunch and my mum and dad for Christmas tea. And then we have our own Christmas lunch on Boxing Day.'

Christmas, for almost all our families, was also a time of increased alcohol consumption and, for 52 (26%) of the women, it was the only time of the year that they bought alcohol for home consumption. Most of our families (138) drank wine with their Christmas meal, and only 15 did not drink any sort of alcohol. This marks Christmas very distinctly from the rest of the year when only a minority of families, 38 (19%), drink alcohol with any regularity in their homes. Practices within most families as far as drink was concerned were similar across the social spectrum: differences in alcohol consumption evident during the rest of the year tended to be minimised at Christmas. This widespread consumption of alcohol was, for most of the families we spoke to, a real departure from normal drinking practice. It is also apparent that alcohol is something that is offered to guests at Christmas time and it is an important part of showing hospitality; in several homes this was the main reason it was bought.

Alcohol is not only *drunk* at Christmas, food is covered in it and cooked with it and flavoured with it. It pervades everything that is sweet, particularly Christmas cake and Christmas pudding. Spirits are particularly favoured, usually brandy or rum, but sherry also plays its part: 'At Christmas time I like to, you know, use quite a lot of brandy in my Christmas cake and sherry in my trifle, you know, I like to make it a bit more festive.' Alcohol adds festivity to food, making it something rich and special; it makes food into a celebration.

Christmas cake, as alcohol, is often available at Christmas to offer to visitors and as such is an important part of the hospitality and generosity with food which is characteristic of Christmas. The majority of our families shared a Christmas cake during the Christmas period, and for most of them it was home made; in 109 families (54·5%), the woman-wife-mother made the cake. Christmas cake was often not eaten for 'tea' on Christmas day but at other times, and frequently on another day. As one woman said: 'This year we had friends on Christmas Eve so we cut it then. So it can be Christmas Eve or Boxing Day because when they've had pudding they don't want much tea.' Christmas cake and alcohol, then, were often available so as to be able to offer hospitality to friends. One friend in particular seemed partial to cake: 'On Christmas Eve when Father Christmas comes we take a piece of Christmas cake and we give it to him.' While drink and cake were offered to friends, however, the Christmas meal itself was confined to and, importantly, defined members of the extended or nuclear family.

The food and drink eaten at Christmas was remarkably consistent throughout the occupational class structure with most families eating roast turkey and drinking wine. This suggests that familial ideology, represented concretely in the provision of a turkey and Christmas pudding for family members who may not come together at any other time of the year, pervades the class structure and at Christmas these practices unite families in all social strata. We would suggest that this phenomenon is an important part of the process of social reproduction of the family as an institution and of familial ideology itself.

Interestingly, there seems to be some class variation in whether Christmas dinner is eaten with members of the nuclear family only or with the extended family. For instance, almost two-thirds of women in occupational classes I/II, IIIN and IIIM shared their Christmas dinner with their extended family compared with just under a third of women in classes IV/V. This, we would suggest, is linked with patterns of family entertaining where there are also class differences (see Chapter 8). Working-class families seem to eat together more regularly as an extended family throughout the year than middle-class families. Thus it is not so essential for working-class families that the extended family eats together at Christmas; cohesion is maintained throughout the year. For middle class families Christmas is more likely to be the *only* time of year when the extended family comes together to share a proper family meal. Thus, although familial ideology is reproduced throughout the class structure at Christmas and finds representation in the consumption of the traditional Christmas dinner, the form that it takes varies with social class.

We can say then that Christmas eating and drinking is marked by the consumption of large quantities of high status food and drink and shows little class variation; the turkey is ubiquitous. The Christmas meal, a proper meal of the highest and most festive status, is also a celebration of the family. Most people eat this meal with other members of their extended family although there is some class variation in this. This practice, however, is common to all classes and indicates that familial ideology, as it is represented in the Christmas meal, is reinforced in every social class each year at Christmas. Thus, as well as being characterised by 'festive' food such as roasts, alcohol and other high status food and drink, Christmas has a special function in bringing together and recreating the extended family. And this ideological function is epitomised in the Christmas dinner, prepared by women and shared by all generations of the family.

The family, however, is not an undifferentiated unit. As we observed earlier, it is characterised by divisions of gender and age, and power and status are differentially attached to people depending precisely upon these categories. These internal divisions are reflected in the preparation and cooking of Christmas dinner, as we have already seen, and in the food that is consumed. Men's preferences are usually acceded to: for instance, one woman never stuffed the turkey because her partner disliked stuffing, and another made custard to go with the Christmas pudding rather than rum sauce because although she liked rum sauce her partner did not. The food therefore reflects relations of power within the family. Generational divisions were also apparent in the food and drink consumed. In 153 (76·5%) of the families, the children ate the same *food* as the adults but in only 42 (21%) did they *drink* the same; the major difference, therefore, arises in children's consumption of alcohol. It was only in a few families that children were given alcohol to drink, and in these cases it was usually just a taste. More usually the children had a special drink, equivalent to the alcohol consumed by the adults but, of course, non-alcoholic. Thus their Christmas drinks were also out of the ordinary but different from those of the adults. So at the same time as uniting families across the social spectrum Christmas food also reproduces gender and generational divisions within families, divisions which are characteristic of the family but which are generally minimised within familial ideology.

Birthday celebrations

Divisions, particularly those relating to age, are also reflected in birthday celebrations, something which again seems to occur within all occupational groups. There is a marked difference between food and drink consumed to mark adults' birthdays and that consumed to mark those of children. In our sample of 200 families almost all the children's birthdays were celebrated with either a birthday cake, at the most simple, or a party of some sort with special party food, at the most elaborate. Adults' birthdays, however, were not always celebrated with food, and, if they were, a special meal of the proper variety, together with alcohol of some description, was much more likely to be consumed than a birthday cake, and none of the adults celebrated their birthdays with special party food.

Of the children 186 (93%) had birthday cakes on their birthdays which were, in 118 cases, made for them by their mothers. The children who did not have cakes were those who had not yet had a birthday (9) and those who were still considered too young to appreciate a cake. Much work was involved in making special cakes for children, cakes in the shape of numbers, cats, trains, houses, and so on, and they were often decorated with multi-coloured icing. Some of the women spoke proudly of these creations and not a few showed us photographs of them:

... they don't seem to like heavy fruit cake very much so I usually make an almond sponge which I do to the customer's request which last year was in the shape of a house. Icing and Smarties on the roof, and a chocolate fence and garden of marzipan and chopped nuts which we do on green shiny paper.

The last one I made was three coloured and I did all round the sides with piping and it did look nice. I put candles on and iced their names on it and put a little decoration on and it went down well. And think if I can bake like that I've no need to spend money at the shop to get it, and it gets eaten. And it's cheaper to do it that way. And I do have pleasure in baking, I enjoy it. I like messing about with the icing set, I like to see the finished article, I'm proud of it.

It was clear that a great deal of loving care and attention went into the making of these cakes; it was part of making the birthday special and demonstrating the mother's affection for her child.

In addition to birthday cakes other food was also eaten in celebration of children's birthdays. Of the children 72 (36%) were given parties with party food; a further 23 (11·5%) had a special birthday tea with members of the extended family invited and 24 (12%) had a birthday tea to which the mother's friends and their children were invited. The women described the sorts of food that were provided at these special birthday meals:

Sandwiches, sausage rolls, tiny little sandwiches, sausages on sticks, cheese on sticks, crisps, I usually bake a birthday cake and decorate it myself. Jellies sometimes, usually bits and pieces.

Sponge cake, little rabbit shaped biscuits, sausages, tiny sandwiches, jelly and ice cream.

The emphasis is on small, interestingly shaped and brightly coloured food that the children will enjoy eating, undoubtedly 'children's food':

I don't do many sandwiches, the children don't seem to eat a lot of sandwiches unless I cut the crusts off, and the tinier the better, they will eat little sandwiches but if they're faced with something quite big they don't tend to eat it much.

Fancy buns and shortbread biscuits which my husband iced and put their names on, he's a bit artistic and he got a paintbrush and colours and put everybody's names on and eyes and noses and things like that.

A family birthday tea was usually composed of food that was suitable for adults as well as children:

Normally either one or both of our families manages to get up and see us and we have a bit of a tea and a birthday cake – nothing out of the ordinary for our tea really, except for the birthday cake and it's always a sponge cake and as long as it's got candles on it they are not bothered. I normally try and do a novelty cake, a shaped one, a train or something like that, trains, boats with ducks on. Last year we had a cat with Smarties and things like that.

It seems that birthday parties and teas with typically children's foods are a particularly widespread way of marking younger children's birthdays; as children grow older, around the age of ten or so, birthday treats and outings become more common. Even between the ages of one and five years we can discern age differences in the way children's birthdays are celebrated. A sizeable minority of children (21%) do not have any special food on their first birthday and where there is a celebration it is more likely to take the form of a birthday tea with cake than a birthday party. Birthday parties are more of a feature of children's lives once they reach around the age of 3 years old – almost 60% of children in the 3 to 5 age group within our sample had a birthday party compared with only 25% of children around the age of 2 and even fewer children aged one. Outings and children choosing their own food do not become common until children are older: we do not have figures for this but it was clear from the women's comments on the birthdays of their older children:

Kate [11] has stopped having birthday parties but she always has a birthday treat, we'll take her and a couple of friends somewhere – sometimes even for a meal, this year we took her to Bibi's with a couple of friends, that sort of thing, we took her to the ballet last year and then they come here afterwards for tea, or before, depending on whatever it is.

Thus the transition from childhood to adolescence and adulthood is marked in the type of food that is used to mark birthdays; at a certain age and stage children's parties and the children's party food that goes with it are abandoned.

Women were very much aware of the distinction between adult and children's food; one woman told us that when her son's grand-parents came round to celebrate his birthday she 'made more adult type food then because it was just a tea. He had a cake, sandwiches and things, but it was just a Sunday tea with a birthday cake.' It is interesting that in some of the women's comments on birthday celebrations there was a distinction being made along lines of gender. Some regarded birthday parties and party food as more appropriate for girls than boys: 'Adam's had two birthday parties. The last one was a nightmare, I said I'd never have another one . . . And I don't think lads are all that bothered anyway, it's more a girl's thing.' We quote at length from the next woman's response to our questions about birthday parties as she clearly articulates the gender differences that many women assume to exist between boys and girls:

Last year for John's, for the boys' party, I did them fish fingers, beef-burgers, oven chips, sausages, fish fingers and oven chips and he had to have crisps as well, he said it wouldn't be a party without his crisps. Then they had the usual jelly and ice cream for a sweet and then I do all sorts of fancy cakes, meringues. [Did he have a birthday cake?] Yes, I did him a Superman. I'm into icing, I like it, I used to go to classes and it was just a long oblong cake and I made a run out of the Superman from his comic in icing and painted it all and iced it and he had this Superman with his cape in blue zooming through the air. We always have a fancy cake. Lucy had a little cottage, that was really nice. It took me about 3 hours to do. I piped it with roses and everything. I love doing it though. [And what sort of food did Lucy have at her party?] I can't quite remember . . . usually things on sticks, you know, sausages on sticks, cheese on sticks. I have little cut out shapes and I do sandwiches in little shapes and they've got no crusts or anything, and put currants for their eyes on ducks and rabbits – they like that. They think sandwiches are sandwiches – they don't like them do they? It's all crisps and that. We always leave the sweet things for after, always have the savouries first and then they'll eat those and then they'll have the jelly and what have you and then I bring the cakes in 'cos otherwise they'll have cakes and crisps altogether and that's all they'll eat . . . They like these little shapes, they like them. It was great at John's they all ate everything, all their fish fingers and all their sausages and all their oven chips, it was really easy 'cos I just put them all in the oven you see so I'd certainly do something like that again. Perhaps hot dogs or something like that next time.

Gender differences were not, however, apparent in the food that was provided for children, although this may reflect an inadequacy in our methodology rather than the absence of difference.

Children's birthday celebrations, as with Christmas food, did not show any significant variation with occupational class. This seems to indicate that the culture of childhood, of which birthday celebrations are an important part, is part of familial ideology and as such exists at all levels of British society. However, the age of the child is significant and indicates that birthday food and the changes that it undergoes mark stages in the child's progress towards adulthood. Once adulthood is reached birthday food changes. Birthday food, and particularly birthday cakes, assume less importance and birthdays are often not marked with food at all. If adults' birthdays *are* celebrated with food it is very different from the food eaten on children's birthdays. It therefore symbolises and represents the distinction between adulthood and childhood much as changes in the food eaten to celebrate children's birthdays represent their progress towards adulthood.

Adults' birthdays, if they were marked at all, were often celebrated by a special meal, usually consisting of high status food with or without an alcoholic drink, and birthday cakes were the exception rather than the rule. Amongst adults gender differences were apparent in the way birthdays were celebrated, reflecting the sexual division of labour within the home and most of the men's greater access to and control over money. Most adults of both sexes celebrated their birthdays with a special meal: 102 (51%) of the women and 109 (54·5%) of the men celebrated in this way. Interestingly, though, 32 (16%) of the men had this special meal cooked for them by their partners, compared with only one (0·5%) of the women, whereas women were more likely to be taken out for a meal by their partners in celebration of their birthdays. This difference, given that most of the women cooked day in and day out with little assistance from their partners, is underlined by this comment: 'Occasionally on his birthday I've cooked him a special treat but I wouldn't think it was much of a treat, I'd rather go out.' Gender differences are also apparent in the marking of adults' birthdays with birthday cake: 46% of men but only 29% of women had a birthday cake. In addition, if a man has a birthday cake it is most likely that his partner will have made it for him, whereas if a woman has one it is most likely that she will have made it herself. Thus women as wives and mothers often bake birthday cakes for all the family including themselves. Many of the women told us that cakes were often baked for adults' birthdays because the children do not regard their fathers (often) or their mothers (less often) as having a proper birthday if they do not have one: 'Oh we often make a cake, yes, for both of our birthdays, more for the children than us really, oh yes, we have a sing-song and blow the candles out . . . not the right number of candles.' Often, though, adults' birthdays are not regarded as important and, as indicated by the comments above, they no longer mark increasing status, reflected in the ever-increasing numbers of candles on the birthday cake, as they do for children. As one woman said:

When you've got children all that sort of goes back to the wall, and it's your kids that are more important, and you make a fuss of their birthdays . . . I don't know, it doesn't seem such an important thing for me really, my birthday . . .

Unlike children's birthdays, occupational class seems to affect the way in which adults' birthdays are celebrated. Women and men in occupational groups I and II are more likely to go out for a meal or have a special meal than those in occupational groups IV and V, and those in the latter groups are least likely to celebrate their birthdays with food at all. The use of birthday cakes to mark adults' birthdays also varies with occupational group. Adults in occupational groups IV and V, particularly women, seem least likely to have birthday cakes, and adults in occupational groups I and II, particularly men, are most likely to.

The fact that adults' birthday celebrations show a variation according to class and children's do not is, we think, significant. As with the food and drink consumed at Christmas, which celebrate the family, particularly in its extended form, children's birthday food is a celebration of childhood, and therefore, along with Christmas food, it plays an important part in the reproduction of familial ideology. Meals out or special meals at home which mark adults' birthdays, or other events such as wedding anniversaries (see Chapter 4), reinforce different social relations and divisions. Rather than reproducing the social unit constituted by parents and children they reinforce the couple relation between men and women. Of course it can be argued that the continuance of this relation is central to the social cohesion of the nuclear family and, in this sense, adult birthday celebrations can be seen as reinforcing another component of familial ideology; one that is based on romantic love and sexual attraction, and which must endure for the survival of the nuclear family.

It is clear from the arguments and evidence we have presented that certain food practices are regarded as essential to 'proper' family life. In terms of familial ideology 'proper' families eat proper meals regularly, eat a special proper meal on Sundays, and celebrate Christmas with the highest status proper meal of the year. These food practices occurring throughout the social structure, serve to reinforce patriarchal familial ideology and, because of this, contribute to the reproduction of the social order. Proper families also celebrate birthdays, particularly children's birthdays, in ways which reflect people's age and stage in the development towards adulthood. These food practices we have picked out as being of central importance to family life. They symbolise the power relations which characterise families, both of age and gender, and they unite families across other social divisions, thus contributing to social cohesion and cultural identity. This is not to say that variation, particularly between classes, does not exist, but that despite this variation the specific food practices that we have been discussing contribute towards the reproduction of the family, in both its nuclear and extended forms, throughout society. Those aspects of family food practices which contribute towards the reproduction of class and other social divisions are explored in Chapters 8 and 9. In the chapters that follow we will concentrate on the way in which food practices within families reflect and reproduce divisions of gender and age: in other words, the contribution of food practices to the reproduction of a patriarchal social structure.

3
Woman's work

In this and the following four chapters we explore the gender division of labour within the families in our sample and its implications for women's relationship with and attitudes towards food.

It is part of family ideology that 'a woman's place is in the home', while a man's task is to go out to work to earn the money to support his wife and children. This very specific division of labour along lines of gender (man the breadwinner, woman the homemaker) is enshrined in policies and practice at all levels of society, from the marriage service to social security legislation. Despite the contemporary rhetoric of equality between the sexes this ideology significantly influences women's experiences, particularly once they become mothers. If equality and an egalitarian sharing of domestic tasks exist between men and women within a household before the arrival of children, and we will explore the extent of this below, it is almost always the case that once children have arrived the allocation of tasks reverts to what comes 'naturally'. That is, it reverts to what is defined as natural within familial ideology; women take on the household and child-care tasks and men assume the mantle of breadwinner. What usually remains implicit in this 'different but equal' partnership is the differential allocation of power which is part and parcel of the gender division of labour. Women, on giving up paid work outside the home, relinquish the power and status that it confers upon them. Their partners, however, unless they are unemployed, retain their status, and the power differential between the sexes is thereby increased.

Women with young children are usually financially dependent on men, they are excluded from the world of paid work, the
work they do within the home is devalued and they are
marginalised by society. Despite this, or perhaps because of it,
they usually shoulder the burden of responsibility for ensuring
their partners and children are well fed and healthy. They take
the day-to-day decisions about food purchase, how much money
they can spend this week, what sort of food will keep the family
happy and healthy. These tasks are women's work. But as we
will show, having responsibility for these decisions does not
necessarily mean that women enjoy power or that they control
the food their families eat. They exercise their power in other
people's interests, above all in the interests of their partners.
Thus although women may have the day-to-day responsibility
for food provision for their families, it is *men* who have the
power and control. Women cook to please men, they decide what
to buy in the light of men's preferences, they carry the burden of
shopping for food and cooking food, but most of them carry out
these tasks within a set of social relations which denies them
power, particularly when they are at home all day with young
children and are dependent for financial support on a man.

Responsibility for cooking

Cooking has long been defined as one of women's major and
most important tasks within the home. Let us therefore begin by
exploring who it is who stirs the cooking pot in families which
include young children. As we have already implied, in the
majority of families in our sample (177 (88·5%)) women were
responsible for the regular day-to-day preparation of meals. In
only 2 families was cooking shared equally between husband
and wife although in about a third of the families men, and
occasionally children, would sometimes cook a meal. Men's
culinary activities were usually confined to the preparation of
non-main meals and 'snacks', a process which was not usually
graced with the term 'cooking'. Apart from the 2 men who
shared the cooking equally with their partners only 23 cooked
on a regular basis, and even in these cases they did not cook
daily or even every other day. And 33 men had *never* cooked a
meal since the couple had been together. Most men only cooked

when their partners were ill or otherwise unable to cook, or maybe cooked the breakfast on a Sunday. This type of cooking is obviously different from the regular provision of proper, family, meals which was what most women referred to when talking about cooking. This remained women's work in almost all the families we spoke to.

Most of the women accepted this division of labour, indeed they felt it was part of their 'job' as a wife and mother to do all the cooking:

He would [help] if I wanted him to as I say but I'm here, it's my sort of job . . . if I'm ill, if I'm dying upstairs he might do a few chips for the kids. He just really doesn't like doing anything like that, he *will* do if I want him to but as I say I don't think he should have to.

And this was often justified by reference to the fact that men worked outside the home and could not therefore be expected to cook. A woman at home all day looking after demanding toddlers, however, could and should.

He can't very well cook through the day, love, 'cos he doesn't come home until ten past five so I can't very well expect him to go and set to and cook a tea, I mean some wives do . . . he'd probably prefer to have me I'd think . . . but he's easy to please, he's not a bit faddy.

Some women, however, felt resentful that they were always the ones to prepare and cook meals:

It's a bone of contention sometimes. He very, very rarely cooks anything. [When does he? What has to happen to make him cook?] Well me refusing to do so is really the only time he will, or if I'm ill, if I'm ill in fact he's very good, he's quite capable of doing so . . . but even if he makes a sandwich he asks you, 'What shall I put in it?' So no, he doesn't. Dreadful really isn't it? And he's not really a male chauvinist either . . . I always blame my mother-in-law for it, his upbringing.

Generally if men did cook they would cook at weekends or when they were on holiday. At these times the rigid sexual division of labour, which most women felt was dictated by the fact that their partners were out at work, could be slightly relaxed. But most men did not cook main meals at all and some were clearly considered to be totally incapable in the kitchen. One woman was asked whether her partner had ever cooked. She replied:

No – can't even boil an egg. When I used to work I'd prepare about 2 meals in one – when I had the time I'd prepare it – and I remember leaving a casserole, you know, steak and kidney and potatoes and everything was in it and all he had to do was get some frozen peas out and put them in. He put the casserole on the top gas which promptly blew up and he put the frozen peas in a pan with no water would you believe. So that's how good a cook he is.

Women often reported that they had to instruct men on every step of meal preparation, or that if they were let loose in the kitchen the mess afterwards was more of an effort to clear up than if they hadn't been involved at all and the women had had to cook the meal themselves. The following descriptions make the situation abundantly clear:

If he's cooking he's only having to cook snacks because it means I'm not here. He wouldn't know how to prepare a casserole. And if I go to work I've got to write on a piece of paper before I go, 'Put the oven on at such and such a time and such and such a temperature', and he should know by now. But I didn't do it one weekend. I prepared it all and I thought I'll just see what happens, and the telephone rang at 11 o'clock at work – 'What temperature do I put the oven on for the casserole? How long does it take?' I was waiting for that phone call.

Well he can cook but I'd rather do it myself because he makes such a mess. When I was first married I went away for the weekend and when I came home I didn't recognise the kitchen, there was fat everywhere. He always cooks everything full blast – he doesn't sort of moderate it or anything – he just throws it in, turns it up high and hopes for the best. He's terrible . . . It's more bother than it's worth, it's twice as hard work if he does it.

Possibly due to this kind of experience some women would not let their partners in the kitchen at all, they felt that it was *their* domain and they wanted to maintain control over it. One man who was present while his partner was being interviewed said: 'Susan doesn't really like me cooking but I mean I have cooked before.' His partner joined in:

I must admit the kitchen is *mine*, I like to use my own cooker and you know I prefer it because I know that if something spills over, alright it's my fault. But if somebody else starts spilling things then I don't like it. But I mean on some occasions when I haven't been well you have done a little bit of cooking haven't you? If I'm late home, say I've got a parents' evening, Robert will perhaps do them a simple meal . . .

This couple were both working full-time as teachers and yet the sexual division of labour as far as food preparation and cooking was concerned was clearly unaffected by the woman's full-time employment outside the home. In fact, our findings suggest that women's employment does not have any effect on whether their partners cook or not, at least at this stage in the life cycle. Those who worked part time were just as likely to be responsible for all meal preparation as those who were full-time housewives. Even the few women who worked full-time did not receive any more help from their partners. They did, however, tend to have nannies who cooked for the children during the day or relied on their parents to look after their pre-school age children.

The nature of men's employment, on the other hand, seems to have some bearing on the extent of their involvement with cooking. The two men who shared cooking equally with their partners were both unemployed and in the other families with unemployed men it seemed that women were less likely to be solely responsible for the preparation of main meals than in other families. This finding needs to be treated with caution, however, as our sample of unemployed families was extremely small.

Social class seems to have more of an impact on men's participation in cooking than either the woman's or the man's employment: indeed, the gender division of labour seems to be mediated in interesting and significant ways which we explore in Chapter 8. Here it is worth quoting an exchange on this topic between one of the women and the interviewer:

I think men should be able to do some basic things like peel potatoes, fry an egg, fry bacon, but most men are absolutely useless aren't they? Really no idea, it's terrible. [I think some try, don't they?] Not in my walk of life. [My husband is not too bad.] Is he good? I wish mine would – you'll have to give my husband some lessons then. I think actually though if you're . . . 'cos you're quite middle class aren't you? I think middle class men are more – they don't think it's sissy do they, whereas working class men think it's real sissy even to be seen washing up. Say if on a Sunday if one of my brothers comes round for dinner well John won't wash up and if my sisters are there he won't but if there's only us he'll wash up whereas if there's anyone else there he won't. It's funny really. I think as I say – maybe middle class mothers are more . . . I don't know but definitely I would say they're more adaptable I think, they're a lot less set in their ideas, you know, I think working class . . . especially men are really stick in the mud, you know. [They tend to be more traditional.] Traditional, the cloth cap image. I think that's true I mean not a lot of them wear the cloth caps – But even with young lads there doesn't seem to be much change from generation to generation – maybe a bit more now obviously but I think they're very traditionalist.

Despite these apparent class variations in the form taken by gender divisions it is still the case that the majority of women in all social classes are responsible for the preparation and cooking of the daily family meal. If men did cook without their wives' instructions it was often not a proper meal that they prepared:

If he said he was going to do a meal he would do something like fried egg, fried bread and fried potatoes which I wouldn't normally do.

Well he never cooks a dinner. He just does something simple, something on toast. He could do more elaborate things but he thinks that's my job to cook, his is to make the money.

This last point is interesting because it underlines the significance of the way tasks are allocated within marriage. If men *were* to share cooking then it would clearly have implications for their undisputed status as the main breadwinner, it would indicate a willingness to discuss and even problematise the gender division of labour rather than accepting it as natural and immutable. However, most of the men ensured that this 'natural' division was not questioned by never, or only rarely, cooking run of the mill, proper, family meals. If called upon to cook they usually relied on sausages and chips or other convenience foods:

Well, like me I can do Yorkshire puddings, roast potatoes and do a cheese pie and all he can seem to do is open a tin of beans or spaghetti. He'll get a few rashers of bacon and chips and a load of beans – ugh!

Clearly this type of food does not constitute a proper meal and men were not expected to be able to undertake this type of cooking. Most of the women felt that this was basically their job and any help they received was a demonstration of the generosity of their partner:

I do more than he does but I think that he does more than his fair share. When I compare him with my father and his father they do nothing, he does quite a lot . . . he'll get the meals a couple of times a week.

If men were involved in cooking proper meals it was usually a rather more special meal that they cooked, such as the Sunday roast or an elaborate meal for a dinner party. It was, however, only a small minority of the men who cooked in this way:

Alan does like to cook, he cooks quite often at weekends . . . When we both worked Alan worked in a branch and he was home before me so he would cook most nights. It's just the convenience really that I'm here, that's the reason I cook . . . He likes to bake, he likes baking and doing fancy stuff. He's not so keen on doing plain things, he finds that boring, he likes all the fancy stuff . . . If we're having a dinner party then he'll cook that, he likes doing that sort of thing . . . he'll sort of go through the cookery books and pick out a main meal, he's quite good at that, he's quite good at organising it all.

Most men in our sample only cooked as a standby or if they were particularly interested in cooking. They were able to choose to cook if and when the fancy took them whereas women had to cook whether the fancy took them or not. But how do women feel about this? Is it accepted as natural and right – the way things ought to be? Is it rationalised as a purely individual response to specific circumstances? Or is it felt to be unfair and resented?

Should men cook?

To try to uncover women's attitudes towards these gender divisions we asked whether they thought it important for women to be able to cook. A majority of them (116) thought that it was important and only a minority (27) felt it equally important that men were able to; an even smaller minority (14) felt that the ability to cook was not important for women. Their responses to this question clearly revealed how intimately bound up with a woman's role as wife, and particularly mother, is the ability to cook: 'Very important really. *Especially* if she's a mother. I can't really envisage a woman not being able to cook . . . You think it's the natural thing, it isn't I know, but you expect it to be.' It also reveals how much the division of labour which allocates the task of cooking to mothers is regarded as something that has to be:

It depends what sort of a woman you are really. If you're going to go back to work after you've had children or if you're not going to have children at all then it's not really important. I think if your husband can cook and you're both working then that's fair enough, let him do it.

But if you're going to have children and give up work you have to be able to cook really.

These two comments stress the importance of cooking to motherhood; the two below link its importance to being a 'proper' wife.

I think it's very important really. I mean we enjoy our food – I don't know quite what Alan would do if I couldn't cook. I don't think we'd have quite married. I don't know how you manage if you can't cook really . . . I suppose you buy it all, convenience type food.

I think it's awful if she can't cook . . . I mean a fella can't do a proper day's work and not come home to a decent meal.

A few women, however, felt that *theoretically* it was no more important for women to be able to cook than for men, although it seemed that in practice they were the ones who *actually* cooked.

Just as important as for a man. I think each relationship, whether married or not, finds its own level. *I don't believe* a woman's role is to be at home and cook and look after the children and her man. Having said that, that is what I *do*, but *purely* because it works out that way.

This type of explanation of gender divisions and their continuation, even when they are not seen as the only or even the most desirable alternative, assumes that women are free to *choose* their role within the family; it is worth noting that the choice made is actually in conformity with dominant gender roles.

Most women, however, saw this gender division of labour as something which was historically and socially determined. It was not something that could be wished away merely by individual women exercising free choice. When asked about the importance of being able to cook one woman replied:

I'd say very important. [Why?] Well to me it's the basic history of the woman doing all that sort of thing and the man going out to work, you know, he's the breadwinner and the wives – I wouldn't say I agree with it that the wife should be at home to look after children, housekeep and cook, but I think it's just the way of the world isn't it really – that's the way it should be.

Several of the women explained the gender divisions within their own households in terms of the way their partners had been brought up:

Well I don't think it's particularly important for a woman to be able to cook as long as one of you can cook. I think it's important for somebody to be able to cook 'cos then you can pass it on to whoever's coming up next. I mean I feel that my husband's lacking in interest and inability to cook is probably a direct result of the way he was brought up.

And another woman's comments suggest that she would probably repeat this process despite her criticisms of it:

Well I've got a theory about this – it's women that bring men up and they bring them up to be bloody useless don't they? They do though don't they? I mean my mother annoys me – I've got two brothers and they're absolutely useless but, you know, we had to wash up and do everything but they never had to do anything and I think that's all wrong. But there again if I had sons of my own I'd probably be the same – I hope I wouldn't be.

There is, therefore, a feeling that it is women, as wives and mothers, who are to blame for men's ineptitude rather than the men themselves. Together with this view goes the opinion that cooking is so simple that anyone can do it, with the exception, it seems, of men:

I couldn't cook, well I never did any cooking before I got married. I think anybody with a reasonable amount of intelligence can manage to knock something together you know . . . people say they can't cook, well it can only be because they haven't tried, I can't see anything very complicated about it you know . . . I think yes you should be able to cook, but there again I can't see why anybody shouldn't be able to cook.

It is common in our culture that women's skills are devalued and not regarded as skills at all. This also happens with cooking, traditionally a woman's skill, at least in the domestic sphere.

Alongside the view, shared by the majority of the women we spoke to, that cooking was an integral part of a woman's role as wife and mother went the view that men should be *able* to cook but should not be *required* to cook in the normal course of events: 'I think men should be able to as well . . . There's always going to come that day when they're going to have to do something.' Women who felt that their own husbands deserved a meal on the table when they came home from work took a different view when they were considering the case of a couple where the man and woman were both working. One woman was asked if she thought that men should cook:

I do – I mean if their wives are prepared to go all day if they're buying a house . . . if she's going to go out all day and he's going to go out all day why should *she* come home and set on and him sit in the chair and wait for it. He could be helping her, could peel potatoes and things like that.

However, even in this imagined set of circumstances it is clearly still regarded as the woman's responsibility to cook; the man is viewed as *helping* her. More usually women thought men should be able to cook in an emergency:

I think they should, yeah, 'cos I mean if anything like crops up, y'know, if like you're in hospital or that. I mean, 'How do you cook mince?' I think there's a certain amount of stuff they should be able to do. I think they could do it if they put their minds to it but like most fellas they say 'Well I've got a wife so she can get on with it'.

And other women thought it would be nice if their partners *were* able to cook just so they could sometimes relieve them of the chore:

It's nice for a man to be able to cook, as well. I mean I would appreciate it if my husband said, 'Oh, I'll do a dinner', you know. He never would, but I know a lot of men that have lived on their own in flats and that have had to or are genuinely interested in cooking, you know. I think it's nice if they do take a turn in it. It's always much nicer to have a meal prepared for you than have to do it yourself – by the time you've fiddled around with it you're not really bothered whether you eat it or not anyway, are you?

A lot of the women's partners were not able to cook even in 'emergency' situations and certainly did not offer to relieve their wives of the chore. Women sometimes felt that they were aiding and abetting men in their helplessness. The two comments below illustrate this point. Usually women going into hospital to have their babies was the one and only occasion on which their partners were left to fend for themselves. Some managed admirably, others did not:

On the Friday before I went in he made sausage, egg and chips but I had to give him instructions. I could see smoke coming out of the kitchen from the chip pan. And when I was in hospital having my daughter he set fire to the chip pan. He lived on Chinese and things like that – I wouldn't mind but I'd made him loads of individual pies and I'd frozen them and I'd said, 'Look, there they are', you know.

He had not even managed to open the freezer to get the pies out while she was away. Another woman's partner was slightly more adept at opening a freezer.

He can warm things up. He can cook his own breakfast. But while I was having Jeremy in hospital for eight days I filled the freezer with meals which I wish I hadn't done, really. I think it's stupid. If I'd thought about it – I was just concerned that he would be eating properly but I think he could have fended for himself really, even down to the shopping.

Even though a lot of the women thought that men should be able to cook they did not necessarily apply it to their own situations, and most seemed happy with this state of affairs, or at least accepted it as just, given that men work outside the home:

I mean a lot of men can cook, a lot of my friends say 'My husband's doing the Sunday lunch today', or something. But it doesn't bother me that John can't. I mean he would try. But you see I'm quite happy if he's looking after the children to go and do the cooking.

I think it's a woman's job, really – maybe you don't agree. I think it's good for them if they can because there's always the odd time when they might have to. I think when they're working and you're at home all day it's nice if you've got a meal ready for them to sit down to.

The ability to cook, and this implies the ability to provide proper meals for men and children, was viewed by most women as vital; it was a fundamental part of women's role as wife and mother. Because cooking is viewed in this way most of the women did not consider that men ought also to cook, they merely thought they should be able to in case a situation ever arose in which they might need to. This view is a long way from regarding cooking as a task to be shared between marriage partners and, as our sample shows, in families with young children a strict sexual division of labour usually operates so that women are the ones who cook. This is rationalised in terms of them being at home all day. But clearly familial ideology has deeper roots than this as even when women are out at work full time they still tend to be the ones who cook, at least in families with young children.

Although men's cooking activities were fairly minimal there were other ways in which they could be involved in 'helping' their partners at mealtimes. During the week, when men were out at work, women did not often expect much help, but at weekends it seemed that men might be expected to lend a hand – at least with the washing up. In fact, men were more likely to take on this task than any other connected with mealtimes; in 85 (43%) of the families men helped with the washing up regularly and in a further 45 (23%) of families men occasionally helped in this way, but this still meant that around a third of the women never received even this form of help. Very few men (7%) helped regularly with actual food preparation, such as peeling potatoes for a meal; around a third (37%) helped with this task from time to time, but half never did so. Even fewer men were involved in the laying and clearing of the table – almost 60% never helped with these tasks: 'Wouldn't help with anything unless I was ill . . . Come to Dave, he works and I do nowt all day so why should he?' Women mostly accept this lack of involvement on the part of men, again justifying it in terms of their work outside the home or their involvement in helping with the children or the garden:

Well I usually say 'Do you want to go and bath the children or would you like to wash the dishes' and we take it in turns. Sometimes I'll say 'You go and pop them in the bath', say on an evening, and I'll start clearing the table and do the dishes, . . . he's very good, he does help a lot.

There was always a feeling of gratitude if men 'helped'. They were doing more than their fair share, they were really 'good'. This again underlines how much it is accepted that these household tasks are women's responsibility and help with them is a bonus and not something that can reasonably be expected: 'He's very good, he'll do anything he's asked, he's not very good at spotting things that need to be done but if you ask him to do something he'll do it.' Some women, however, were not totally reconciled to their situation and resented their partner's lack of co-operation. One woman, when asked if her partner ever helped, told us:

No; full stop . . . he doesn't sort of see the need for washing up pots and drying them, even when I ask him he's usually got some excuse. He won't thank me for telling you this but it's true. No, I always do the pots myself and cook myself so that's that.

She wasn't entirely happy with this state of affairs:

I often have a grouse about who's going to do the pots afterwards 'cos I'm not one for getting up and doing them immediately, they quite often get left till the following morning which annoys me when I have to get up early. I know sort of if I've not done them it's my own fault but – I'm quite ashamed of it really. But I get so tired in the evenings sometimes I feel 'Oh I can't take that', you know.

If women worked in the evenings this made it more likely that their partners would do the washing up:

Well I go to work you see at twenty past five and he always washes up afterwards which is quite good. He'll lay the table if I ask him.

This was not, however, always the case, as one woman described:

Well what used to happen is I'd cook the meal and have it all ready and we'd sit down and eat it, I'd go to work and I'd come back and the pots would be left for me – which they are always left for me when I come home and I either do them when I come home or the next morning . . . I got quite fed up of this at one stage so I said 'Right you can cook the tea then'. I feel awful saying to cook the tea but when I'm working . . . That's how I got it changed over you see 'cos I thought bugger it he can cook it and I'll wash it up after.

Obviously some men are prepared to change the gender division of labour to a certain extent if their partners make an issue of it, and it does seem that if women work outside the home men are more likely to help with mealtime tasks, although not, as we saw earlier, with cooking itself. Those women who were full-time housewives were much less likely to receive regular help from their partners than were women working outside the home, whether part-time or full-time. For example, over half the men married to women who were in paid employment helped with washing up on a regular basis (3 of the 4 men married to full-time and 54% of those married to part-time workers) compared with a little over a third (38%) of men married to women who were full-time housewives. However, apart from washing up, which appears to have become something most men do from time to time, it is a minority of men who are involved in these tasks. Meals, their preparation and all the work they involve, remain largely a woman's domain despite the impact of women's employment outside the home.

Work patterns are obviously crucial to this division of labour. Men being out all day was cited time and again as the main reason why women did all the cooking and why men could not be expected to take their share of these domestic tasks. This is emphasised by the changes that take place, although fairly minimal, when women are also working outside the home, and by the observations made by women about the increased involvement of their partners at weekends or during their holidays.

Clearly in most of the families men were conspicuous by their absence from tasks connected with food preparation and clearing away after a meal. And when they were involved they were helping their wives. In other words, the chores were the women's responsibility and the amount of help they received with them depended on the good will and availability of their partners. Most of the women we spoke to accepted this division of labour with little criticism, particularly if they did not themselves have work outside the home. All the tasks associated with food and mealtimes were accepted as part of being a full-time wife and mother; a change in the gender division of labour might become part of the family agenda when women worked outside as well as inside the home.

Children and cooking

Given women's views of the root cause of men's inability to cook and lack of interest in cooking, it is interesting to look at their attitudes towards the participation of their own children in cooking and food preparation. One of the women graphically described her own father's lack of cooking skills when she was asked if she thought men should cook:

Oh I definitely think they should be able to do something because my dad is the most useless person at cooking. If anything happened to my mum my dad would live on cornflakes I think. He's awful, he can't – no I won't say he can't – he won't be bothered to do things for himself. When my mum goes to work she leaves him a sandwich for his lunch and if it's cold she does him soup, a packet soup. Well a packet soup you have to boil for 5 minutes or whatever – now she has to boil it for that 5 minutes so that he can just heat it up because he wouldn't be bothered to wait for 5 minutes. *I think boy children should be taught at school how to cook – I think it should be compulsory that they are taught how to look after themselves.* (Our emphasis.)

This sort of attitude seems to indicate that although men's participation in cooking and other mealtime tasks is minimal, that of their sons will be altogether different. However, our evidence suggests that although a number of women subscribe to these sorts of views, the majority are bringing up their children in conformity with the dominant gender division of labour. Socialisation of children, at least as far as food is concerned, is differentiated along lines of gender.

We talked to the women about the ways in which their children helped in the kitchen and from these discussions it became clear that attitudes towards children's help depended very much on gender, even when a conscious attempt was being made to move away from these stereotypes.

Baking was the most likely form of food preparation for children to participate in and was often regarded as play. It was also seen as an appropriate occupation for boys *and* girls; after all, it is a game rather than the serious matter of feeding the family:

When I bake he always lends a hand. He will always weigh the flour, he'll scoop it out of the big jars and things and put it onto my scales . . . and roll the pastry out . . . help me bake cakes and stir things. And whisking, he'll sometimes hold the handles of the mixer and mix things for me. It's just to keep him entertained as much as anything. (Son aged 3 years.)

They help with baking – it's fun for them to cut out the shapes. (Sons 5½ and 3½ years.)

Some women noted differences between their boy and girl children in the amount they helped and often there is a clear attitude on their part that it is more appropriate for girls to help than boys:

Stuart (4) shows more interest, *he should have been a girl.* I love to bake and he's the one that's in the kitchen wanting to do it . . . but Sarah (7) keeps out of the kitchen, she keeps out of the way. (Our emphasis.)

Emma sets the table ready for me and she'll – when I've done the vegetables she usually puts them in the pans for me. The boys don't do anything but Emma helps quite a lot.

Emma's brothers were positively discouraged by their father from helping in the kitchen:

He doesn't mind them playing in the kitchen he's a real chauvinist – he likes a man to be a man and he doesn't like anything like that particularly . . . They play in the kitchen but they will never help like Emma does . . . (Boys 1½ and 4, girl 7.)

Several women mentioned that their daughters were more helpful than their sons. But, in these cases it is difficult to assess whether this was due to their sex or their age, as in other families with two children of the same sex the younger one often seemed inclined to be more helpful. However, if the younger more helpful child was a girl women often gave their sex as the reason for their being more helpful:

Sue's more interested . . . If I start washing up she'll say, 'I'll dry for you mummy', and she'll pull the chair up and dry the pots for me so she's good, she's more into – well I suppose she's a little girl, she sees what I do . . . But Martin won't, very rarely will he help me but I don't mind I just – sometimes I get mad with him, I'll say 'Look will you fold your clothes up?' (Girl 4½, boy 7½.)

Some women consciously tried to ensure that their sons and daughters helped equally: 'As they get older I'll want them both to help, I had to help my mother and Gilbert had to help his mother.' (Girl 3, boy 1 year 8 months.) Interestingly, even when women seemed to want their sons to learn to cook, differences emerged in the way that they spoke about girls and boys. One woman was asked whether she would teach the boys how to cook when they were older. This was in the context of her description of her partner's total inability to cook:

Yes. Our Mark (9 years old) – they do a certain amount at school now when they get older and Mark will help. Say if there's something he wants to do then I'll do it with him but I think they should know how to look after themselves yes. [What about Rebecca (2 years old), is it something you'll encourage her to do?] Oh yes. She sits on my work top and holds the mixer now and things like that now. Oh yes I shall definitely teach her to cook properly – if she has a husband like mine she'll need to know.

This difference in treatment needs no comment, particularly when the ages of the children are taken into account. But it indicates the influence school can have on attitudes and practices regarding cooking. Another woman also mentioned this:

Yes they'll lay the table if I ask them to and they're quite good at clearing away. Julia occasionally likes to cook and Sam does cooking at school so he will experiment at home from time to time. (Boys aged 14 and 4 years, girl 8 years.)

The event of boys learning to cook at school was regarded positively by all the women whom it directly affected.

Women's attitudes towards their children helping varied. It seemed clear that most children, given the chance, enjoyed joining in tasks in the kitchen, but while some women let them help others found their help to be more of a hindrance than anything else:

She's just starting to take an interest. If I'm in the kitchen she's got to be in the kitchen. If I'm at the sink she's got her chair or stool at the sink – she loves it if I do any baking 'cos I let her slop it around a little bit or I give her some pastry to play with. She'll wash the dishes only I have to go and wash them again 'cos she's not done them properly, and she gets water all over the floor and down her sleeves and everywhere, but I don't stop her. They like to play with water so I let her do it. (Girls 3 and 1 year).

They do try but, I know it's awful, I get impatient and I do tend to tell them to get away. I feel a bit rotten afterwards. I mean they've got to learn haven't they? (Girl 3, boy 1).

A number of women mentioned that the kitchen was a potentially dangerous place for toddlers, particularly as far as cooking was concerned, and very few children actually helped with meal preparation:

I try and keep him out of the way because he tends to reach over the cooker to see what's in the pans and I don't like that. The kitchen is only small so it could be dangerous (Boy 4, girl 7).

Some women also didn't insist on their children helping because they felt that they would have enough to do when they were older:

I ask, they don't do it off their own bat. They will take their own plates out and put them in the kitchen and I'll say 'Who's going to do the washing up?' If I didn't say anything they wouldn't do it. It's a thing I've never pressed and I think it's because I'm not bothered. They like to go out and play so as far as I'm concerned they can go. They will do plenty when they get older so I don't stress it to them at all. (Daughters 11, 7 and 1.)

This usually only applied to women's attitude towards daughters!

It seems clear from these comments that there are differences in the amounts that children helped in the kitchen, and that these differences relate to the age and sex of the children and the attitudes of the women themselves. Gender seems to be an important factor in determining whether women and men

encourage or discourage their children from helping with
cooking and other domestic tasks. It also seems that most very
young children are enthusiastic about joining in with these
tasks whether they are girls or boys; it is only gradually that
they learn which tasks are appropriate to their gender.

Responsibility for shopping

Shopping for food is another task which is defined as women's
work within familial ideology and the vast majority of women
we talked to did all or most of the food shopping. Of the women
92 (46%) were wholly responsible for the food shopping – they
shopped for food on their own. Only 3 of the men did the food
shopping on their own. In 21 (10·5%) of the families men and
women shared the food shopping, either taking it in turns to
shop or doing it together, and in 82 (41%) of the families the
women did most of the food shopping themselves with some help
from their partners. This sort of help was usually driving women
to the supermarket for the main shop, looking after the children
in the supermarket aisles, or buying the odd item of food from
time to time.

Given this sexual division of labour over food shopping, it is
not surprising that the majority of the women – 170 (85%) – said
that it was they who decided what food was bought, while most
of the others said that they made these decisions in consultation
with their partners and children. It was not only the women who
did all the food shopping on their own who decided on what food
was bought, for even when men participated in food shopping
their involvement tended to be tangential rather than central.
Typically, they provided the transport and helped carry the
shopping; they pushed the trolley or helped to look after the
children; and occasionally they made individual forays down
supermarket aisles for items already decided upon by their
partners. One woman, whose husband took her in the car to the
supermarket, described this typical pattern:

I think because we have three kids he's more or less keeping them in
order and if I'm going to queue up at the cheese counter I'll say to him
'Will you get the yoghurt?' or whatever. He's sufficiently in touch with
what we are getting to know what I'm talking about. If he went by
himself without a list I think it would be fairly chaotic – if I give him a

list it's fine so long as I'm fairly precise. To him if I said 'Sugar', I would have to specify type and amounts. So mainly he's looking after the kids, pushing the trolley and occasionally we split up to get different lots of things.

Women, then, usually drew up the mental or literal list of what was to be bought and this was true even in those few cases where men did all of the food shopping. This is because shopping is, of course, intimately connected with cooking; the person who cooks knows what they require and what they have in stock: because men were rarely involved with cooking they were rarely aware of the range of foods required or of the various ways in which they might be prepared. This meant that items usually had to be specified in detail when men shopped for food:

My husband will go, but you have to write down *everything*. He goes to the supermarket, you've even got to write down where they are – he's just not that way involved, I don't think, he's just not interested in it . . . if ever I've been ill and I write a list I've got to write down the *brand* of things that we get.

Understandably this led some women to feel that, as with cooking, they were better doing the job themselves. But, of course, women's expectation that men could not shop on their own initiative itself contributed to a situation in which men very rarely became efficient shoppers. Furthermore, there is some evidence that women preferred to do the shopping alone. In part, this was because shopping tended to be seen as one of the more pleasant household tasks; some women had few other opportunities either to get out of the home or indeed to spend money. As one woman whose husband never did any food shopping said:

I don't really want him to either . . . I enjoy it, and I don't want him to take over. There's a certain amount of pleasure for me, shopping. I haven't lost the thrill of going into town to shop, y'know. Silly, really, isn't it? I like spending money, whatever I'm spending it on, I enjoy it.

Other women, however, felt that they could get the shopping done more quickly and efficiently if they went alone:

If I go by myself I know what I want and get what I want, whereas if he's with me I tend to say 'Shall we have this?' or 'Shall we have that?' and I don't get a very good response from him. It doesn't work at all. I'm much, much better myself, I can think what I'm actually doing. Actually he quite enjoys going but as I say I prefer to go by myself.

And men were often reported as suggesting or picking up food which women did not consider necessary; indeed, husbands were often blamed by the women for buying food which they had not intended to purchase:

He puts things in the basket that I wouldn't normally. You know, I can go to the supermarket and get just what I want, just what I need, but he can't he has to buy all sorts, biscuits and cakes.

We'll end up spending more than I would if I didn't have him with me. He goes 'Let's have some of this', 'Let's get some of that' but he does help, yes.

This sort of impulse buying created problems for women budgeting on a low income. In general, it must be emphasised that most men did not appear to be interested or keen food shoppers. Achieving a more egalitarian division of labour for food shopping appeared to some women to extract too high a cost in terms of both time and expense, while for others it was clear that men could not or should not be expected to share in shopping.

   Although women were in the main the ones who decided on what food was to be bought, shopped for it and then cooked it, this responsibility is not necessarily accompanied by power and control. The social relations and gender divisions of labour within which these processes take place reveal that women's responsibilities are very circumscribed. It is, in fact, men who, both directly and indirectly, wield the power; women's own interests are subordinated to those of men. This subordination is explored in greater detail in the next chapter: here we wish to relate it to the gender division of labour within the families we spoke to as we think it is important to place women's responsibility for the purchase and provision of food in this wider context.

The effect of paid employment

As we have already pointed out, the vast majority of women took daily decisions about the food that was to be bought and eaten by their families. The most important consideration in this process was the preferences of their partners and children; they had to buy food that was liked and would therefore be eaten

by their families. But although women took these daily decisions, it was far more frequently men who decided on the
amount of money that would be available for food expenditure.
In fact, in fewer than half the families did women have the power
to decide how much of the total family income would be spent on
food. This was the case in 44 families where women managed all
the money and in 40 families where money was managed jointly
by both marriage partners. In the other families the men took
out their own spending money, which was often an unknown
amount (to the women), before handing over their wages (39) or
gave their wives a housekeeping allowance (52). In 5 families the
men managed all the money, even going shopping with their
partners in order to be able to sign the cheque, and in 20
households other arrangements which could not easily be
classified were made. Clearly, however, the systems of money
management adopted by the families we talked to meant that
while women organised and carried out the food shopping, they
had to work with a set amount of money decided on and handed
out by their partners. In a large number of families it was
therefore men who controlled food expenditure although women had the responsibility of carrying it out on a day-to-day
basis. This, we would argue, is responsibility without control
and is a very real demonstration of the unequal relations of
power existing between men and women.

There is some support from our material for the conclusion
that the power enjoyed by men results from, or is at least
reinforced by, their participation in paid employment outside
the home. At the time we spoke to the women most of them were
at home looking after very young children. Those who did work
in paid employment usually worked part-time or nights so that
they could combine child-care with work outside the home. This
picture contrasts strongly with the occupations of women
before they had children when, almost without exception, they
had been working full-time outside the home. (See Table 1.1,
Chapter 1, for details of women's occupations prior to the birth
of their first child.) However, most of them had had to give up
work once they became mothers (it is important to note that this
decision was often not made through choice) and if they
managed to find work to fit in with the needs and demands of
their children it was often of a lower occupational status than

the work they had been doing previously. This is particularly true for women who had been doing secretarial or clerical work before they had children who often took jobs as cleaners or worked in a pub because the hours fitted in with their child-care responsibilities. With the exception of the four women in full-time employment, who were all professionals in the sphere of education, the women's work was characteristically low paid.

Most of the women's partners were, by contrast, in full-time employment, they were the ones who were bringing home the wherewithall to keep the family alive, they were, indeed, the breadwinners. In fact almost all the women 175 (87·5%) said that their partner was the main breadwinner while 7 (3·5%) said they were joint breadwinners. Only 2 women regarded themselves as the main breadwinner, 7 of the women lived alone and a further 9 regarded themselves as having other sorts of arrangements. This situation clearly reflected the women's lack of status in occupational and financial terms and contrasted quite strongly with the situation that had existed prior to the birth of their first child. Even then 113 (56·5%) of the women said that their partners had always been the main breadwinner. A typical response to this question was:

It's difficult to say because we always knew that one day we'd want a family so we always lived off his income, his income always paid the bills, mine always paid the one-offs, 'cos at that time we were busy collecting our furniture and buying a car and things like that, so I suppose really we've always lived off him.

Women's wages are, realistically, regarded as impermanent if couples intend to have children; when that happens they will usually have to do without her income. But prior to this event there had been much more variety in the gender division of labour: 11 (5·5%) of the women had been the main breadwinners, fairly often while their partners were students, 55 (27·5%) of the women had regarded themselves and their partners as joint breadwinners, 3 women had lived alone and 18 had either not lived as a nuclear family or had not responded to this question. Thus the arrival of children had pushed many couples into adopting a more sharply demarcated gender division of labour. Most of the women became financially dependent on men because they gave up their paid work to have children, and if men had previously shared some of the domestic tasks like cooking this also changed. Several of the women commented on this:

He used to do more when I worked full-time . . . it's me being at home you see.

When I was working full-time he finished work earlier than I and I usually left prepared what we were going to have and when I came home it was ready.

He used to cook a lot before we had Peter and I was working but now he doesn't seem to cook as much because I'm at home all day and it doesn't really bother me.

However, almost half of the men (93 – 46·5%) had never cooked regularly even when their wives were working full-time outside the home and only 7 couples had shared cooking equally. Men's cooking was almost always sporadic and took place if their partners arrived home later than them or if they were ill. Even then it was not always the case that men cooked: 'I used to begrudge coming home, I used to get home later than him, and I didn't like going into the kitchen while he was sat down waiting for me.' Clearly, cooking, for most couples, had always been regarded as the responsibility of the women, and even those few couples who had shared cooking equally before the arrival of children adopted a much more rigid gender division of labour once they became parents. This did not always happen without resentment and regret, but even if women felt like this their partner's job outside the home was usually regarded as just cause for their not cooking or sharing other household tasks. One woman felt that because the woman is 'the one who gets lumbered [with cooking] . . . it helps if you are good at it and enjoy it'. She went on:

At the moment I feel Graham's quite bogged down with his job and everything and I'm quite – I suppose I'm coming to terms with the fact that I'm at home all the time – whereas we used to share it and now I do it all and, I feel as though I *should*, but I do resent it a bit – that he can't help me so much. I don't expect him to because I think he's got enough to cope with just holding a job down really.

Often the type of food cooked also changed, partly because women had more time to spend on cooking and partly because they had less money. Instead of steaks or chops, which were quick and easy to cook on returning from work, stews and casseroles were made. As well as taking longer to cook they were usually cheaper. As one woman put it:

I suppose with being working it was things for quickness like we'd buy chops to grill, steak to grill, rather than doing casseroles – more tinned vegetables, I buy more fresh vegetables now, tins of fruit for pudding and things like that.

So leaving paid work and having children has a profound effect on women and the gender division of labour within the family. It means that cooking and providing food assume much more importance for women, it takes more time and they have less money and more people to feed. Food provision moves to the centre of women's lives and, at least for the years while their children are at home, most of their waking hours are devoted to thinking about and preparing food. It is a constant preoccupation and it is clearly felt to be an important part of being a 'good' wife and mother. What are the implications of this for women? How does it affect their relation to men and children, their views on food and health, and their relationship to their own bodies? These are the issues that we wish to explore in the following chapters.

4

Women and men

Women cook and provide food for others. For the women we spoke to those others were primarily their partners and children for whom they cooked on a daily basis. In this chapter we want to concentrate on the significance of food in the relationship between women and their partners. We want to look at the emotional investment made by women in food and its implications for family eating: the way men's food preferences are prioritised and women's own preferences are neglected. We shall argue that the gender division of labour within these families renders women's position less powerful than that of men, and that the way food is distributed between men and women reflects their relative status. Women, as servers and providers of food, usually prioritise other people's needs over their own. They sacrifice their own preferences to such an extent that when asked about their own likes and dislikes most of them replied that they would eat anything; they fitted in with the rest of the family: 'I like to please my family more, I mean it doesn't matter to me, I can eat anything.' In contrast, when they ⅄ were asked about their children's and partners' likes and dislikes, they went into great detail describing them. These responses indicate the significance of cooking for others, their preferences take precedence over women's own. Indeed, if women's preferences take precedence they feel selfish and guilty.

I don't get anything to cook that I don't like myself. That's very selfish isn't it? My husband loves broad beans but we never have them yet we've got loads in the freezer – but the children don't like them and I don't like them and we're not cooking them just for Paul.

Food was seen as playing an important part in maintaining the couple relationship, in expressing affection between partners and in ensuring that men remained happy and contented with their wives. This was evident in differing ways in different relationships and appeared at two distinct levels. Firstly, the level of special meals or gifts of food, events which did not occur on a daily or even a regular basis, and, secondly, the level of daily food provision. We will first of all explore the more unusual events and then look at the significance of daily food provision for the relationship between women and men.

Food's emotional significance

Food was clearly invested with emotional significance by women. The preparation of a man's favourite food was regarded as a way of 'treating' him or a way of making up after a quarrel. Food, on these occasions, is a demonstration of affection and care. One woman, when asked if she ever made special food for her partner as a treat, replied: 'Yeah, usually, when we've had a quarrel I try and make it up. If Daddy gets something nice he'll say, "What have I done?".' She went on to describe the food she had cooked the last time this had happened:

I tried a new recipe with pork in cider and that was nice, it wasn't too expensive either because the pork was quite reasonable and cider as well is not too expensive and we had a big gallon container of cider left over from when we went to Devon, so the most expensive thing it had in it was the cream which was to thicken it – cream is one of those things that's a bit expensive but I tend to – if it says use cream I use the top of the milk, but I did actually buy cream for this.

And another woman said that she prepared her partner a special meal: 'If I've been a bit grotty – I can be sometimes. I suppose we all can can't we? If I'm feeling a bit guilty about – 'cos you always take it out on the nearest don't you which you shouldn't but you do?' Food – particularly in the form of a special meal such as that described above, something which is out of the ordinary and has taken more time to prepare than usual – expresses emotions. Women demonstrate their affection through this type of special meal. One woman articulated this very clearly in a way which, though untypical, points up the emotional significance of food. She was asked whether she cooked special food as a treat for her husband and replied:

Yes I do . . . I cooked him a Chinese meal last week. I try, I do try and recognise very hard to produce every night for him something that is not simply run of the mill. I remember meeting a woman when I was in hospital . . . a 60 year old woman who was some kind of sub-aristocrat and had been married to someone from the BBC who had led her a horrendous dance, and she said that it had been important to her to always live in a state of love with him and that the preparation and presentation of nice meals on a nightly basis was one way in which she could express what she felt for him. I remember being very impressed by that and, up to a point, I try to create that in my life with Peter.

Most of the women did not express themselves in this way, but this does not necessarily mean that they were not making similar kinds of emotional investment in the food they prepared for men.

Sharing a meal with their partners without the children was also a feature of many of the women's lives. They would prepare a special meal, set the table in a way which was more elaborate than usual, perhaps including candles, and share this meal with their partners after the children had gone to bed. One woman said: 'The one special meal we have is on a Saturday night, and that's a regular thing. I think everybody should have one night when they have a good meal, a bottle of wine and all the trimmings.'

Wedding anniversaries or other events, such as the birth of a child or success in a job interview, could also be celebrated by the preparation of a special meal. One woman spoke about the way she and her partner celebrated their wedding anniversary: 'We're getting less romantic as the years go by. We used to always go out to dinner, but now sometimes we just give each other something we need, or go to the pub for an hour.' This comment points up the fact that sharing a special meal together is 'romantic' in that it symbolises or recreates the couple's relationship to each other. A meal out together or a special meal at home after the children have gone to bed holds an important place in maintaining the initial relationship of love and sexual attraction between partners. This type of meal is usually more elaborate than normal, family meals. It may have two or three courses, is often accompanied by wine or other alcoholic drink, and frequently involves a special setting of the table to mark the occasion as different. But this type of meal also involves more expense than a normal meal and this probably helps to explain why this practice seemed more common among middle class couples than others. And time was also needed to prepare this more elaborate type of meal and with small children around this is often in short supply.

I used to, I can't now, I'd love to do. I often used to do it for special birthdays and things, things I really knew he enjoyed then I would make prawn cocktails to start with, a full three course, I used to love doing that, and a special sweet . . . we'd have a bottle of wine as well . . . but now he'd probably turn round and say we haven't got the time or – he puts me off a lot more than I would – I would probably try and do things myself but it would mean palming the kids off on him while I got cracking, or else eating at 9 or 10 o'clock at night which is really too late.

Because of exigencies of time and money these elaborate meals *à deux* were not a common feature of most of the women's lives. However, affection and caring were expressed through food provision in other ways. Many women bought or cooked food for their partners that was not eaten by other members of the family:

I occasionally get him things that he maybe wouldn't think was a treat but things that I know he likes that I don't like like cod roe, you know, I mean they're not dear but . . . or crab he likes and I don't like it, so I do odd things like that, I wouldn't say they were any dearer but it's things he likes and he eats on his own.

I sometimes do a curry for him on a night for a treat; they [children] won't eat it. Or I sometimes make him egg curry pie for his pack up.

So often men's preferences were catered for in this way, as a way of 'treating' them. But also women gain pleasure from providing food that is enjoyed. As one woman put it: 'I think that if I make a special effort to make something nice it is appreciated – put it that way – and I'd probably partly do it because I know it would be appreciated.' It was very rare in our families for men to prepare and cook special food for women. If men 'treated' women with food or used food to demonstrate their affection it usually took the form of buying sweets or chocolates or, more rarely, taking them out for a meal. This happened, if at all, on women's birthdays or, more usually, on their wedding anniversaries. In fact, many of the women, when asked what they would consider a treat for themselves, told us a meal out would be a treat because they would not have to do the cooking:

Anything that anybody else cooks. I like to go out and eat for a treat, I don't really mind what I eat, it's just where I eat it, I like somebody else to have got it ready completely and somebody else to have the washing up to do.

Some men did go to the trouble of making their partners special meals and when this happened it was very much appreciated. It was however an extremely rare occurrence. One woman recounted the meal her partner cooked for her to celebrate the birth of their first child.

I'd just had Philip and he bought me a new dress, and he made me sit in the room one night with a glass of cider and he said, 'you can't go in the kitchen', and I didn't know what on earth was going on, he'd never done it before. When I went in he'd done steak, mushrooms, tomatoes and the lot, and a bottle of wine, and he said that was for having Philip.

Giving a gift of food to one another was also fairly widespread amongst our families; 107 of the men and 81 of the women gave food as a gift to each other. And many others treated themselves by buying food which was slightly out of the ordinary such as special cakes: 'We tend to go shopping on a Saturday and bring cakes back just as a sort of treat, it's just something we do really, we have a cake on a Saturday morning.' Chocolates were often exchanged as gifts: 'Either of us might buy it for the other one and then eat it, share it.' But when women were slimming, as many of them were, flowers often took their place! Chocolate bars might be brought back by men for themselves and their partners if they had been out: 'He often brings a Mars bar or something home because when he's out he stops for petrol and he often buys a couple of, well, Twix or something you see and then he brings them home . . . he generally just brings two, one for each of us, and we have them later on.' Chocolates could also be invested with an apology, a way of making up after an argument. 'He buys me chocolates but you can't really call that food can you? Occasionally, if we've had an argument he may come home with a box of chocolates which always surprises *me*.'

The dominance of men's tastes

The use of food in these almost *conscious* ways as an expression of feeling, whether it be affection of repentance – or just 'togetherness' – was comparatively rare amongst our sample.

What was far more common, in fact so common as to be taken for granted, was the concern for men's well-being shown in the regular, daily provision of meals. Whether this symbolises affection or the unequal relations of power within families is arguable. But it is clear that women take men's food preferences into account to a far greater extent than those of their children or themselves when they are planning and preparing meals. We asked the women what factors they took into account when deciding what food to buy for the family and 146 (73%) mentioned their partner's food preferences; 126 (63%) mentioned their children's preferences but only 90 (45%) mentioned their own preferences. It seems that men's preferences have more of an impact on what women cook than those of any other family members. Why should this be so? Why should women prioritise men's food preferences over and above everyone else's? To provide an answer to this question we need to explore the implications of the fact that it is women who shoulder the main burden of food preparation and cooking within families with young children. And that, as we remarked at the beginning of this chapter, women cook for others. This is not a simple statement, for women cooking for others means that they cook to please others. They cook to ensure that people are well fed and well looked after, to ensure that those who they cook for firstly *eat* what is provided and secondly *enjoy* it. The ability to provide food that is good and that is appreciated by a hungry family, particularly a hungry man, is a fundamental part of being a wife and mother. And enjoyment of cooking for most women depended on the end product being enjoyed by others. Their own enjoyment was secondary. Several of the women talked about their enjoyment of cooking in terms of providing for an appreciative family: 'I enjoy putting a nice meal in front of the family and seeing them enjoy it. I've always got pleasure out of that. I think that's the main thing.' She went on to say that if her partner was away: 'I don't enjoy it. I don't enjoy cooking it as much or eating it – I don't really enjoy it without him. It's funny, isn't it?' Food that was not eaten was a waste, not only in terms of the food going in the bin but in terms of the time and effort that had been wasted in its preparation.

This need for the end product to be appreciated perhaps goes some way towards explaining the dominance of men's preferences in terms of the food produced. Women felt hurt and rejected, in themselves, if the food they offered to their partners was refused. Children's refusal of food was not usually taken so seriously as they were expected to have changeable tastes and food fads. This partly explains why their preferences are not taken into account to the extent that men's are.

Many women told us of events, usually when they were first married to or living with their partners, which involved a partner's rejection of food. And many referred to a process of trial and error through which they learnt what foods their partners would and would not eat. This process, and the need to provide men with food that they liked, was part of the taken-for-grantedness of most women's lives. This woman's experience was typical. She was asked whether she cooked different food when she was first married.

Much the same – I'd maybe do the odd prawn cocktail and scampi and chips when we had more money. But much the same because it was what Mark was brought up on. I did try the odd spaghetti bolognese and such but he didn't like it so it wasn't worth trying anything new at all. I've won him round to the occasional curry – I love that but it's got to be my own – if he can see me putting the best stewing steak into it he'll eat it then.

Indeed, women seemed to expect to have some problems with their partner's tastes when they first started cooking for them, and regarded themselves as particularly fortunate if men always ate what was put in front of them: 'Well you don't know their likes and dislikes do you? Just the basic dinners even – like roast beef and yorkshire pudding – you've got to try it to see if they like them which *I was lucky you see* because he liked everything' (Our emphasis). As well as finding out what foods their partners would accept women often went through a period of cooking elaborate meals: this seemed to be a way of celebrating the fact that they were together as a couple: 'Well I tried everything, I really went to town when I first got married, and put weight on . . . I don't know, you try to please don't you when you first get married.' This often wore off due to pressure of time or money or, as the comment above indicates, an increase in weight! This was commented on by one of the women:

Oh yes we had prawn cocktails to start with and pork chops with apricots and sweets, and, Oh God!, we put loads of weight on. I think to start with you cook to please each other and it's like a social event every night when you've both been out at work, and money was more available then than ever it is now.

All these comments underline the importance of pleasing the man you are cooking for. There is concern to cook meals that he will eat and enjoy and discovering his preferences is part of becoming a 'good' wife and showing that you care for him. Several of the women also felt themselves to be in competition with their mothers-in-law: they would try to emulate their cooking or try to wean their partners on to their own, superior cooking. If women try and please through cooking the food men prefer then men can also please by expressing preference for their partner's cooking above anyone else's – *particularly* their own mother's. This comparison can sometimes cause ructions:

He'll say, 'Why don't you try this like my mum does?' and I feel like saying 'Well get your mother round here and do it!' – But he will say things that his mum does and I will try, if that's what he likes. I don't like fish in a sauce, I prefer it in batter or breadcrumbs, he likes it steamed and his mum does that in a nice white sauce. He likes it so I will do that for him but at the same time I'll put mine in breadcrumbs and fry it – I don't like steamed fish.

A corollary of the process of eliminating the foods men dislike from the diet is subordinating your own preferences, and this almost always occurred if conflict was to be avoided. One woman was unable to cook anything other than very plain dishes for her partner:

My husband is very traditional-minded about food, he doesn't like anything Chinese or foreign, he doesn't like anything with herbs in it apart from salt and pepper so I tend to stick to the same thing most weeks – I rarely buy anything just for myself . . . I'd like to buy salmon for myself which I don't buy now. I get tuna occasionally. I'd like to eat all sorts of food, foreign foods, but I don't bother; as I say it's too expensive to buy a tin of it just for myself so I forgo it.

It will be remembered, though, that if men like foods that no-one else in the family likes women often buy and cook them specially as a treat. This is not so likely to happen the other way round, although one or two women mentioned eating foods they themselves particularly liked if they were alone at home. One woman treated herself in this way:

I have a passion for spaghetti and butter, that kind of thing, which nobody else in the family likes, so occasionally I do that sort of thing when I'm on my own, so I have a curious notion of what's a treat. For me a treat – personally for a treat it's anything which I like and nobody else in the family likes – kippers for one and spaghetti with butter on and that sort of thing. . . . That's much more of a treat than sticky and gooey buns – everybody likes those.

In fact, in many families women bought and cooked food for their partners that nobody else would eat: 'I buy liver . . . that's something I don't like and the children don't like but my husband does so I buy liver for him and we probably have omelettes.' And here the situation is reversed: 'I like liver done in the oven and he doesn't, he doesn't like liver – so I just don't bother doing it for myself.' The dominance of men's preferences within the family's diet is made clear by this woman's experience:

My husband had quite a lot of fads when we first got married you know, he wouldn't touch certain things or he won't eat them a certain way or that's it. Obviously that's influenced over the years. What gets eaten and what doesn't. It's funny that if he decides that he wants to experiment with something it's quite acceptable whereas if I do it he'll say, 'What the heck's that?'

Her partner mainly liked 'a roast and things like sausages and, you know, things like meat cooked in the traditional way rather than continental.' And he disliked 'what he calls sloppy food, he won't consider at all – spaghetti or pasta or anything like that, he just says "Forget it!" ' She, on the other hand, liked 'curries and things like that.' This situation seemed to be fairly widespread with men expressing a preference for a proper meal of meat and two veg; good, plain home cooking. In other words, they often exert a conservative influence over families' diets and prevent their partners from experimenting with food or introducing changes into the diet.

Men had various ways of making their views felt. Some were very cautious, as one woman told us: 'I used to make quite a lot of pizza and after about seven years he told me politely that he didn't like it very much so I didn't make it any more. He didn't say anything for all that time.' This was extremely unusual. Most men were not so accommodating. The woman whose husband would only eat plain food recounted the following experience.

If I cook something that's got a whiff of herbs in it or something he'll put his knife and fork down and say, 'I'm sorry but I'm not eating it'. Occasionally he'll get through it but I have known him to refuse to eat it and maybe go and have a biscuit or a piece of cake instead. [How do you feel about that?] Not very happy. He usually waits until my parents come and I've prepared something a bit out of the ordinary and he'll leave it. I'm not happy but there again I'll not make a scene, I'm not one for rowing – I'll go off and have a little weep to myself. It's all over, I mean we never argue much about anything like that and then he'll probably say sorry and eat it next time but the next time I know better and don't put it in you know.

It should be said that it was not a majority of the men in the sample who had at one time or another refused food: 130 (65%) had never refused food or had only refused it if they had been ill. However, this does not necessarily mean that they will eat anything they are presented with: it often means that their partners have very successfully adapted the diet to their preferences as this woman told us.

I cook what I know he will like. Even if I cook something different I make sure the basic food is what he likes. I mean I don't try things knowing he won't like them. Things like pasta I know he won't eat that, so I don't cook it. But he's never actually refused anything. He might get it thrown at him if he did.

There were, in fact, no reported instances of women throwing food at men, but a small number of the women reported that their husbands had thrown food at them if it hadn't met with their approval. This violent rejection of food was an extreme reaction, but it underlines the relations of power which underlie the gender division of food provision. Women within this relation are subservient and subordinate, they are the servers and providers of food for men. We will quote at length from one of the women's accounts as it gives a very clear picture of the power relations governing food provision. During this interview both husband and wife were present. The husband began by saying:

There was once where you made something I didn't like – I remember that.
Wife: 'Oh yes, I forgot about that.'
Husband: 'Yeah – But apart from a broken plate and a rather dirty wall there was no other damage.'

Wife: 'I forgot about that altogether.'

Husband: 'Yeah, I threw it at you didn't I? Do you remember?'

[Did you?]

Husband: 'Yeah. Oh dear me, I think I said something like, "Shove that fucking muck" – Oh, sorry the tape's on isn't it? I don't want to be rude. That was when we'd just got married wasn't it and you thought that was an acceptable standard of nourishment.'

Wife: 'I thought it was nice, it tasted nice.'

[That was right at the beginning of your marriage?]

Husband: 'That's right, yeah. She's never given me any of that rubbish again so that's all right.'

It is hardly surprising, in view of these responses and the hurt experienced by rejection of food, that women try to cook according to their partner's tastes in food. One of the single-parents had found divorce a liberating experience because of this and was now free to vary her own and the children's diet. Her partner had been fond of 'fry ups' and 'greasy' foods. She told us:

He didn't like cheese and potatoes, whereas I do potatoes with cheese in and they love it, the children love it and I love it. 'I don't want that, I'm not having that.' He wouldn't have food that wasn't heavy food, you know? He liked solid food on his plate – he wouldn't have salad and none of this noodles. That's not good enough for a working man.

Many of the women reported their husbands as refusing to eat salad, particularly if it was presented to them as a main meal on their return home from work.

I used to buy fresh meat, vegetables, potatoes, fresh greens, just a meal. Unless I do a meal like that he won't class it as a meal; if I do a salad it's not a meal to him . . . I've just got to do a meal with meat, vegetables and potatoes . . . he expects a hot meal and I think he deserves it.

Men expect a proper meal on their return from work and women seem to feel that this is what they deserve and is appropriate for a working man.

The importance attached by women to the provision of a proper meal for their partners was brought out when we asked them if they would cook differently if they were living on their own. Only 25 of them said they would continue to cook the same, the others would all change their diet to a greater or lesser

extent. The main changes that would occur seemed to be a
reduction in meat and a move away from proper meals.
Additionally some women said that they would no longer get
any enjoyment from cooking and for this reason would not
bother: 'Don't think I'd bother just cooking for one – I mean I
never do if they're not here. Perhaps have sandwiches. I don't
think there's any point in just cooking for yourself, I'd rather
cook for somebody else.' A reduction in meat would often be
balanced by an increase in other foods, foods which are not
normally considered to be part of a proper meal such as soup,
fruit, cauliflower cheese, and so on. One woman told us: 'Left to
my own devices, if I was living on my own I would probably live
on soup, milk puddings, muesli and fresh fruit. I'd eat a lot less
meat and a lot more fruit and vegetables.' And the main reason
for providing proper meals for their families was often men's
insistence on meat. 'Well we eat quite a lot of meat and I'm
prepared to have say two or three days without it . . . I'd be quite
happy with cauliflower cheese you see but Michael would
regard it as a vegetable, not the main part of the meal.'

Men also felt that they should be provided with a proper meal
on their return from work. A meal that consisted of lower status
meat such as bacon or fish fingers was not considered appropriate by either men or women as the following comments
illustrate:

A man that's been at work all day doesn't want to come home to fish
fingers. He wants something a bit more substantial.

A couple of weeks ago I gave him bacon and he said he was sick of
seeing bacon – we'd only had it a month before – it's not as if he's having
it every night. He don't consider bacon's good enough meat y'see. It's
expensive as everything else really but its more breakfast to him. I'd
made the bacon with potatoes and cabbage.

Women also feel that there is some truth in the saying that the
way to a man's heart is through his stomach. In fact, a minority –
85 (42·5%) – of the women we spoke to felt there was no truth in
this saying, the others (apart from 5 (2·5%) who did not know) all
felt there was at least some truth in it. Their responses to this
question suggest not that food is used by women as a means of
manipulating men, but that provision of food which is preferred
and enjoyed is a way of ensuring that men are happy in their role

as breadwinner and a demonstration that women are fulfilling their role as wives. For women who are financially dependent on men, as was the case for all but 14 of the women we spoke to (4 working full-time, 10 single parents), the loss of the male breadwinner would have severe consequences; keeping him happy was partly to be achieved through feeding him well. One woman put this into words:

I think so. I mean if you didn't cook, if you didn't give them what they liked and wanted, they'd go out and buy their own or go to somebody else I suppose. Yeah, I think it's true that the way to a man's heart is through his stomach, I've always said that.

It also ensures that men are able to work: 'If they have good food they can work better. If you get a man that's not had a proper meal and that he's going to be miserable isn't he? . . . I'd say it is quite true.' And shows that they are cared for: 'It shows that you care in a way doesn't it? . . . if you show you've put some effort into it and some thought, then it makes them feel sort of wanted.' Some women felt that anybody felt better for a good meal, but a greater number thought that this was more true of men than women. One woman who thought there was not really any truth in the saying went on: 'Well I say that but I think men like to eat well. I think generally most men enjoy their food.' [Is it different for women?] 'Generally I don't think women are as bothered.' As one of the women pointed out to us this saying is itself sexist. It assumes a specific gender division of labour in which women are subservient to men and part of their role is to keep them well fed and contented. A woman who does not do this, or who does not think it is important, is not properly fulfilling her domestic duties. However, the majority of the women we spoke to accepted this division of labour, even if they did not altogether agree with the form it took. One woman, for instance, told us that her husband often refused the food she prepared for him: 'He likes all his vegetables mushy and now and again I like them half-cooked, there's more goodness in them that way so now and again I do them like that and he'll leave them.' This domineering attitude clearly irritated her and she went into great detail about his male chauvinism when asked the question about the way to a man's heart.

Oh yeah. That's how I got him [laughter!] I think it is yes actually. I think a lot of men look for a woman to how their mother is. 'Cos I mean I run about after him really a bit silly at times. If he won't hang his clothes up I'll hang 'em up. At one time I left them for a week and they were just piled up. I nearly drowned in the pile. And he says, 'You'll get sick of this before me', and I did . . . I think a lot look for a wife that's like their mother . . . I mean if they didn't like your cooking they'd be always at the fish shop or somewhere like that – or round at his mother's.

All these factors mean that women tend to cook food according to their partners' preferences on a daily basis. So that, really, men are pampered, their tastes are catered for in the very way that a family's diet is structured. As one woman, who said she never 'treated' her partner with food, put it: 'I know the things he has more of a liking for and I class a lot of that really as every day but usually, two or three times a week, I'll do the stuff that I know he likes best.'

Food distribution

The privileging of men was also evident in the distribution of food between women and men and between boys and girls within our families. There were certain foods which enjoyed a higher social status than others. This became clear from the women's accounts, especially when they were talking about the foods they would eat for a treat. We have already mentioned meals eaten in restaurants in this context, but it is important to look at what such meals might consist of. They usually contained a high status meat, such as steak, alcohol, cream and pudding or gateau. A working-class woman described a treat for herself: 'A nice fillet steak with mushrooms and chips, and after that a nice big piece of gateau, and then one of those coffees with cream on top – Irish coffee, and cheese and crackers.' She would drink brandy with this type of meal. Sweet foods were often treats, particularly if they were not eaten regularly. Chocolate, cream cakes and 'sticky, gooey' puddings were all mentioned by the women when they spoke about the foods they would like to buy but were unable to afford. Comments such as, 'I'd buy a nice piece of meat for a treat – beef – we never, ever have beef, apart from special occasions – Christmas!' were legion.

These sorts of responses indicate that certain foods are associated with pleasure and are highly valued in social terms, at least within the dominant food ideology, which most of the women we spoke to accepted. Within this ideology meat, particularly red meat, enjoys the highest status. As we have already noted, meat was viewed as being especially important for men and red meat, particularly, carries connotations of virility and male sexuality. We only have to think of the number of steaks eaten by male heavyweights before a fight to understand the strong connotations it also has of male aggression and strength within western culture. Meat, therefore, is a food which, while enjoying a high *social* status, is particularly associated with men: it carries sexual connotations. White meat is considered to be a less 'strong' food. Consider, for instance, the distribution of chicken meat: men are often given the drumsticks, the dark meat, while women and children eat the white meat. Thus, foods seem to have an association with sexuality and gender: some are viewed as 'strong', 'masculine' foods while others are 'weaker' and more 'feminine.' The contrast between red meat and white meat is the most striking example of this. Alcohol, a drink associated with pleasure and celebration, is also associated with masculine culture, usually masculine pub culture. Its consumption has in the past been regarded as a male preserve. Men are expected to drink in large amounts whereas women are not; we have only to think of the ladies' glasses which are still provided in many pubs to recognise that these attitudes persist. And as well as being associated with men alcohol, especially wine and spirits, is associated with pleasure and celebration. Sweet foods are also ranked in their own hierarchy, although in relation to meat and alcohol their status is not high. Cake, particularly the ceremonial cakes associated with Christmas, weddings and birthdays, enjoys the highest status and puddings or desserts enjoy a higher status than biscuits and sweets because of their association with the proper meal. However, this rather depends on the type of pudding: a carton of fruit yogurt or Angel Delight clearly does not occupy the same position as a sherry trifle or gateau, both of which – importantly – contain cream and/or alcohol. Biscuits and sweets are also eaten between meals and this may partly explain their lower social status. Cakes and puddings have a place in even the most elaborate types of meals.

This brief description of key foods associated with pleasure and social status throws some light on the very marked gender division of food distribution within the families in our sample. We show the average consumption over a 2 week period of these food items in Table 4.1. Here we are, of course, drawing on the women's diary records. High status meat includes such meat as steak, joints of meat, chops and fowl; medium status meat refers to mince, bacon, stewing steak, liver and kidneys, and low status meat includes meats that, according to the women, could not be included in a proper meal. These are such things as sausages, luncheon meat, meat paste, beefburgers and so on. These categories do not take into account all the gradations of status within meats, but they give a broad indication of the relative social values attached to different types of meat. The other categories are self-evident. The averages presented are averages of the *frequency* of consumption and do not relate to the *quantity* of food consumed at any one time. This method is likely to *under*estimate gender differences and we discuss this further below.

Table 4.1 *Frequency of consumption of certain foods during diary fortnight*

	Adults		*Children under 12*	
	Women	*Men*	*Girls* (168)	*Boys* (124)
High status meat	4·5	4·9	3·0	3·2
Medium status meat	6·8	9·0	5·0	5·7
Low status meat	5·1	6·8	5·0	5·6
Cakes	6·7	7·3	4·9	4·9
Puddings	7·0	7·0	9·3	9·3
Biscuits	8·0	6·4	11·1	11·5
Sweets	3·5	2·6	8·2	8·0
Alcohol	2·7	4·4	0·2	0·2

If we look first at the figures for women and men we can see that average consumption of all types of meat is higher amongst men than women. The women's accounts suggest that men's greater consumption of high status meat is either the result of the fact that women sometimes cook special meals for their husbands alone, as a treat or because men disliked the food which was being offered to the rest of the family. Men might also be given the left-overs of the Sunday joint in their Monday 'pack-ups' to be eaten at work. Similarly, men were often offered the left-overs from meat meals as additional 'snacks' or given them in preference to the non meat meal the rest of the family might eat the next day. Men's greater consumption of low status meats seemed to be the result of their eating such food as snacks and suppers – in other words, as additional rather than inferior meals when compared with other family members. Interestingly, when we look at children's consumption, although there is by no means the same strong contrast between boys' and girls' consumption of meat as that which pertains between men and women, similar gender based patterns of consumption are evident. Men, and to a certain extent boys also, are therefore privileged in their consumption of that high status food, meat.

Turning to sweet foods, we can see that once again men are most likely to consume the high status food – in this case, cake. The main source of this inequality seems to be the practice of reserving cake left over from Sunday tea for men's packed lunches; sometimes women even bake cakes precisely for this purpose. Biscuits and sweets, on the other hand, are of low social status and are consumed more frequently by women and children than by men. This can partly be explained by the fact that their consumption constitutes a break in the day for women and children at home, but it does not eliminate the fact that the sweet food of highest status is reserved for the male bread-winner. The status of the consumer is reflected in the status of what is consumed. In this sense we can speak of men as being privileged in terms of food consumption: not only are their preferences given priority but they consume higher status foods more frequently than other family members.

Alcohol exhibits a very clear gender linkage among adults, again with men consuming it far more frequently than women. This pattern is not evident amongst children, but then in most of the families children never drank it. They might be given the odd taste if they asked for it, but only one or two children drank alcohol, and then it was usually wine very diluted with water. If a gender pattern exists it was not possible to perceive it from our data. However, among adults alcoholic drinks were clearly associated with men; yet another instance of something with a high social value being consumed more frequently by men than by women. It is interesting to speculate – although it can only remain at the level of speculation – whether the high social status attributed to certain food and drink arise because of their specific association with men, or whether it is their high social status which leads to a situation in which those with most power – whether within the family or wider community – monopolise those commodities for their own consumption. Clearly in the situation we are describing it is women who actually distribute the food according to these gender-based patterns. We would agree with Delphy (1979) that this is an instance, and a very important one, of women having internalised their own subordination to such an extent that it is seen as 'natural' and 'inevitable'.

Food needs

This process of normalising and naturalising men's greater access to foods of high social status takes place largely through ideologies of food needs which prioritise biological difference as determining that men and women have different, biologically given, food needs. The women talked about food needs and from their accounts it appeared that men were always assumed to need more than women. This was usually justified in terms of men's greater physical activity than women at work, and in terms of the 'fact' that men are bigger than women.

It was not only in terms of frequency of consumption that gender differences were apparent. Women also indicated in their diaries that they gave larger helpings of food to their partners, larger pieces of meat, more potatoes, more sandwiches and so on. This was accepted as natural. Comments such as, 'Of course, he's a man, he'll eat more won't he?' indicate that men, merely by virtue of their sex, were bound to eat more than women. Some women realised that this was not necessarily always the case.

It's like I suppose you always tend to give a man a bit more food than what you're having and sometimes you find that the bloke would rather have had the smaller plate and the woman the larger one. I think a lot of people think you should give a boy more to eat than a girl, and a man more to eat than a woman.

Many of the women's reasons for giving their partners larger helpings than themselves could certainly be justified in terms of men's greater involvement in strenuous, physical work. But many could not, and these justifications were still advanced when the men patently did not need to eat as much as they were doing. One woman, for instance, gave the following account:

He seems to need a lot more. No matter how much I give him to eat he'll always have a cake or a biscuit afterwards, even if we've had a pudding he looks around the house to see what's going. He's got a very good appetite. He does a heavy job, he's a fitter, so he works outdoors and indoors, he's got a manual job and I think that gives him more of an appetite. I think that's probably what it is, because well, I'm indoors.

This contrast between men working outdoors and women working indoors recurred again and again, and seems to be an important distinction between men's and women's supposed physiological requirements. However, what on the face of it may seem an entirely reasonable set of statements becomes somewhat problematic when we contrast it with what this same woman said about her husband later on:

My husband has put over a stone on this last year, and his shirts are like that now. I said to him really you should be more careful. He eats good and then he still looks round for something else. When summer comes I shall do more health foods for him . . . he's big but it's just a middle age spread. If he goes to work in the car he doesn't have any exercise but I'm on the go indoors so I maybe burn more up . . . When I do cut him down he complains and wants more – he goes and gets some cakes or something so he's worse off.

It appears then that the indoor–outdoor distinction is more of an ideological construct than a dichotomy that necessarily reflects a real differential in energy requirements between men and women. For instance, a woman whose husband was not a manual worker justified his need for more food than herself in terms of his work being outside the home: 'Well he's more active, he needs more I think . . . . he's out and about – I'm quite housebound I'm afraid.' The fact that he went out to work was itself seen as producing a need for larger quantities of food. Work carried out inside the home did not carry the same connotations; it is women's work and – by definition – it does not use up energy or make women tired! When women discussed children's food needs it also appeared that they were assuming that boys would be active and use up lots of energy *outside* the home while girls would be quieter and less active *inside* the home: 'I think boys need more 'cos they burn a lot more up don't they, they're more active I think, then as they get older with football and everything.' It was partly the different activities that boys and girls become involved in that justified their differential food requirements, and partly girls' interest in slimming once adolescence is reached. This was mentioned by many of the women as something which would lead to girls eating less than boys, and it was very much tied up with notions of sexuality and body image. One woman put this very clearly:

I think boys always have hearty appetites, according to what people tell me – I think a lad will probably tuck in more than a girl because I think girls probably get more conditioned towards the slimming bit whereas boys, I don't think it would enter their heads.

And considerations of weight and body image were often paramount in women's minds when talking about differences in food needs, even when they appeared to be critical of the commonly held view that men need more to eat than women. One woman was rather indignant that we even asked a question about differences in food needs. She said:

I need more than he does, I expend more energy per day than he does, I mean he works pretty hard and he's racing about in his car. But I think I probably use more energy in an average day. And I've got a big appetite, I always have had, *that's why I haven't got a waist and my stomach sticks out further than it should as well.* (Our emphasis.)

For women large body size is unacceptable, slimness is the goal, whereas for men the standards are different. They are *expected* to be bigger than women. As with the comment above, if women feel themselves to be the wrong shape, too 'fat', the reaction is to cut down on food, to try to reduce their body size. With men, on the other hand, their large size is itself often used as a reason for them to eat more than women. One woman's comment is typical: 'I give him bigger portions of pudding, he's got a bigger appetite than me, he weighs more and he's fatter so he needs a bit more really.' Different standards are applied to women and men. Apart from any considerations of actual energy expenditure on work, whether inside *or* outside the home, men are expected and permitted to be larger and heavier than women. Cultural standards for men's and women's body sizes are clearly different, but most of the women related these differences to 'biological' factors such as metabolic rates, energy requirements and so on, even, as we have seen, when their partners were overweight and in sedentary occupations. What we wish to point out here is the ideological definition of differences between men's and women's food needs. This definition depends as much, if not more, on cultural stereotypes, as it does on actual energy requirements and physical size. As one of the women put it:

They probably end up doing – boys end up doing manual work and girls end up doing office work, and boys probably tend to eat – from what I've seen – a lot more; they tend to do a lot more outdoor, athletic type things and I think they have healthier appetites. But I think given that they are given a non-sexist upbringing and education obviously their needs are . . . [So it's not an actual basic need?] No I don't think so, I think it becomes a need because they come to need more because physically they grow bigger and they're healthier and they've been given more and I think it's a social thing really that becomes a physical thing.

Women clearly see their role as one of refuelling men with food so that they will be able to return to work well fed and full of energy. Central to this process is the regular provision of proper meals, including that food most necessary to the male, meat! Men's involvement in work outside the home, and their financial support for women and children at this stage in the life cycle, mean that they are highly valued family members. They have more economic power than women and children and this situation is reflected in food provision and distribution. Women's main role is to provide their partners with food, in a form which is appropriate and acceptable, and which demonstrates that they care for the wellbeing of their partners. In extreme cases, if the food provided is not appropriate male reaction can even become violent, a clear demonstration of the unequal power basis of this relationship. The distribution of food between men and women, and the dominance of men's food preferences within the family's diet, is therefore an outcome of the gender division of labour. Food also carries a heavy emotional significance. Sharing a special meal together is a pleasurable experience which reinforces a couple's identity, whereas displeasure in food can produce conflict and considerable hurt. Given women's situation of dependence, both emotional and financial, on men, particularly at this stage in the life cycle, the privileging of men in terms of food provision is hardly surprising. Indeed, it is a symbolic representation of the subordination of women within the family, a concrete expression of their position as servers and carers of men.

5

Women and children

Food occupies a significant place in relationships between women and their children, and the sorts of foods which children consume and the manner in which they consume it tell us a great deal about age relations within the family. In the previous chapter we illustrated the importance of food as a concrete indicator of gender relations. In this chapter we are going to explore the relationship between parents and children as it is revealed at family mealtimes, the role played by food in mothers' care of their children throughout the day at home, and the way in which children's food differs from that consumed by adults.

The contradictions of family mealtimes

As well as cooking the proper family meal it also falls to women to ensure that mealtimes are a happy family occasion. This often proves to be a delicate balancing act requiring them to subordinate their own needs and desires to those of their partners first, and their children second. It is part of familial ideology that families are safe havens free from contradictions and conflict. Women, isolated in their homes with young children and cut off from the experiences of other women, often feel under considerable pressure to reduce to a minimum any conflict that might arise at mealtimes. They attempt to do this by balancing the needs of their children against the needs of their partners, and somewhere in this process women's own needs become totally submerged. These conflicting demands and pressures on women are particularly acute because of women's feelings about men 'deserving' a proper cooked meal on

the table on their return home from work, the importance of
feeding children properly, and children's assertion of their own
likes and dislikes. Men's needs and desires usually took
precedence: 'My husband's home at 10 past 5 on a night and I
like it on the table – give him a chance to wash his hands – and
on the table. I don't like him waiting for it. I mean he's been at
work all day, he's entitled to his tea.' The need to strike a
balance between these often contradictory demands often
results in meals becoming very tense occasions as the following
remarks illustrate:

It's chaos. I think it's a very tense time really because he comes in tired
and he's been at work all day and I am very short tempered me and
they're clinging round me and they're running around me for bits. If I
ever left them it would be at tea time – I would walk out of the door and
I'd say, 'That's it' and they could get their own. So I would imagine with
my children it would be – that is a real strained time for me. As I say
she's only maybe an hour and a half off from going to bed so she's like
this and she knows if she tugs at me long enough I'll give her a biscuit
and they're rooting and I could – it really gets – I can have a lovely day
but I could shout at him as he walks through the door some days, you
know, which I suppose he must feel the same. Once we sit down it's OK
but it's trying to dish out and strain all the pans with her about – I think
I'm that busy watching what she's doing I tend to pour it over my hands.
It is nerve racking.

Men are not only felt to need a proper meal on their return home
from work, it is also imperative that mealtimes be made as
pleasant as possible for them when they are tired and hungry.
However, mealtimes also provide the opportunity to teach
children to eat properly. What this implies is that they learn to
eat a proper meal, using a knife and fork, sitting at table. In most
of our families children began participating in family meals and
sitting at table between the ages of 18 months and 2 years. It was
clear that this participation was an important part of the
process of making the child part of the family. It is also an
important part of the process of socialisation and involves the
exercise of control over the child by the parents in order to
enforce conformity with accepted patterns of behaviour at
mealtimes. The importance of controlling children's eating was
often brought out when women told us of the changes in meals
that had occurred once children started participating in family
meals. Some women had changed the time at which the main

meal was eaten and some had changed the place, now eating at table whereas before they may have eaten in front of the television.

Before Timothy came along we used to eat every meal on a tray in front of the TV, and it's not comfortable to eat that way, you don't really realise it until you stop doing it. But I don't want Timothy to think he can just whiz off into the living room with a meal on a tray and eat on the floor or in a chair. I like to eat at the table.

Often the type of meal being consumed dictates whether control is necessary. For instance, one woman said:

If it's sandwiches or anything like that we sometimes have those on our knees. If it's anything where you use a knife and fork or if there's fruit or anything that can be a bit messy, they sit at the table. It is harder to control them when they're not at the table.

Clearly, the felt need that children eat a proper meal 'properly' necessitates control over them, and this control is easier to exercise if they are sitting at table. However, children do not necessarily submit to this and conflict often arises because they refuse to eat the food that is provided, preferring other things such as chips and fish fingers, archetypically 'children's' food within British culture. The refusal of children to eat proper meals can therefore be interpreted as a challenge to parental authority. It reveals that the proper meal is consumed within social relations of power, power exercised by parents to control children's behaviour and to socialise them into socially acceptable behaviour.

Conflict at mealtimes rather than peace and harmony seemed to be the norm within our sample; only 55 of the 200 women reported no arguments. In 120 families parent-child conflict was reported and in 39 families there was conflict between the parents. The nature of this conflict reveals not only that adults exercise power over children but that there is a power differential between husbands and wives.

If we look at women's accounts of tension at mealtimes it becomes clear that there are often disagreements between themselves and their partners over what their children should or should not eat and that they, very often, have to take avoiding action to minimise the chance of conflict and maintain the authority of the father in the family. In some situations conflict is not avoided and then it becomes clear that a power struggle is in progress. This struggle reveals what usually remains hidden. One woman, whose husband insisted on her providing him with a meat and two veg meal every day, told us what happens if the children don't want to eat and her husband is present: 'If there is an occasion when the children don't want to eat something I don't force them but if my husband's here he forces them and that causes a terrible row.' She was asked, 'Between him and the children?' and replied: 'It starts with him and the children and then I start sticking up for the children, if I think he's said too much to them, so the argument's between me and him. I don't believe you should force them – they will eat if they want to eat it and I know whether they like it or not.'

In many families the father's word carries more weight and women acquiesce in their partner's decisions even though they may not agree with him; they accept his dominance. This power relation is learned by the children through the provision and consumption of the proper meal. One father made his son eat some peas at a meal. His wife's tactics would have been different, but she wouldn't display this insubordination in front of the children.

Now I'm not saying that I would have done that but he sat at the table with him until he'd eaten all the veg. I mean I never go against what Mark – I mean if he tells them to do something I never say 'Oh, don't make him do that' but personally I wouldn't have made him eat it.

She went on to say that even if the children left something that she knew they liked she wouldn't insist on them eating it. They would just have to do without until the next meal. Her approach avoids the need to persuade or force a child to eat food:

Say if they left half their dinner on a Sunday that would be it, they wouldn't get anything else 'cos I know that they like – say it was roast pork I know that they'll eat it – so it's their hard luck if they leave it, they'll wait till tea time.

But when her husband is present the proper meal is eaten by the children according to the practices laid down by their *father* rather than their *mother*. The consumption of the entire meal was something that was obligatory if the father was present, but not if he was absent, a clear indication of differential power and authority within the family. This woman's experience is similar:

'If we're at table – as far as eating the meal I don't argue with him, if he doesn't agree with something I just keep my mouth shut . . . if he says something I let it go whether I agree with it or not.' She was asked whether her partner did the same if she said something and replied: 'He wouldn't *argue* with me. I usually say the wrong things. He would stand by me if he agreed but if he didn't agree he would say something whereas I would just shut up and wouldn't say anything.' Again in this family the woman reinforces her partner's authority in relation to the children whereas he may undermine hers, a lesson about gender relations which children take in with the food they consume.

Of course, not all men acted the part of Victorian patriarch; not a few were reported as being softer with their children than many women allowed themselves to be. Sometimes women, worn out by the needs and attentions of young children during the day, were given a break by their homecoming partners who, arriving relatively fresh to the task, found greater reserves of patience and humour with which to coax food into reluctant young mouths.

He sort of pulls faces at them and makes them open their mouth that way. 'You open your mouth like Daddy' and, you know, straight in. Sometimes they make animal noises and car noises and it's chugged into the mouth this way – it amuses them and it does work.

But it does seem true to say that in general women tended to defer to their husbands' authority when conflict arose at mealtimes. Whether men were easy-going or strict in their attitudes to children's behaviour affected the whole tenor of family mealtimes.

This inequality in the power and authority of marital partners can lead to bizarre arrangements. One woman went through a phase of feeding her children before her husband came home from work in order to minimise the risk of conflict. Their ideas on feeding their children differed.

He has a firm idea of three set meals a day more than I do, but then he's not at home with the children all day, every day, that tends to – it doesn't matter how much you sit down and say I am not going to let them have things between meals . . . you eventually come round.

This view of his had given rise to arguments in the past.

The only times we've ever really had arguments is when the children were a lot littler and he wanted them to eat a proper meat and potato dinner and they didn't want to eat a proper meat and potato dinner and I'd be more inclined to say, 'Don't force it down'. The times he did it used to aggravate me intensely – was when I'd put little piles of separate things on their plate and I'd think that if they don't want to eat the vegetables they might eat the meat 'cos there's no contact with the vegetables, Jon would come along and, 'Come on eat it all up' and spoon it all together . . . But they are eating a lot better now so we don't have that sort of argument . . . if you start arguing over mealtimes what hope have you got?

Jon's insistence that the children eat a proper meal had led his wife to take avoiding action which she described in some detail.

She wouldn't eat so many things that there was no point trying to sit us all down, four of us together, and have a proper meal because I knew she wouldn't eat it which would have inevitably led to conflict between Jon and I . . . I saw it as a phase of some sort and that eventually she'd get through it which she has done . . . so I did purposely, I gave them their meals and said that they were tired and 'I'm doing so and so for us later' just so I knew that what I gave her she'd be able to eat and he wouldn't see that I was giving her chips every night . . . I let them have their meals just totally separately and I just gave them something I knew they would eat.

For a period of time this woman abandoned the consumption of proper, family meals altogether so as to avoid conflict. But in most families their consumption, even by very young children, is regarded as an important daily event, and through gradual or forced adaptation to the consumption of the proper meal children are socialised into the social order as it is reflected in the family and accept the system of power relations that characterise it. The methods by which this end is achieved are various and in some families it is achieved more thoroughly than others.

Children and 'proper meals'

But why is it that children refuse proper meals and yet they will eat 'children's food', breakfast and the non-main meal with relatively few problems? Most of the women reported their children's eating as being problematic in some way and it became abundantly clear that most of the problems arose from their reluctance or outright refusal to eat food provided in the form of a proper meal. There seem to be two main aspects of this, firstly, that children wish to be independent and, secondly, that refusal of food is often a rebellion against parental authority. The child's wish to be independent and to act autonomously from his/her parents is made difficult by the proprieties associated with the proper meal. Knives and forks are difficult to handle, meat needs to be cut up and it is difficult to chew, food cannot be picked up by a child in its fingers. This all means that a child has to be helped and cannot eat independently. Food in other forms is easier to manage as one of the women pointed out: 'He likes bacon sandwiches. Don't you James? Because you can eat those on your own. He's going through a phase where he doesn't like things fed to him so they must be in some form that are easy to eat.' The food eaten for the non-main meal or breakfast is much easier to eat than a proper meal. Sandwiches and toast are eaten with fingers, breakfast cereal is eaten with a spoon. In addition to this children have much more choice over what they eat at these meals whereas they have little choice at the main meal of the day. They can also exercise a certain amount of choice over the sweet course of a main meal. One woman described these differences.

Andrew at midday [the main meal] has what he's given. Some days he gets a choice of what there is for pudding, you know, if I've got two or three things available at teatime I always ask him what he wants and in the morning usually because sometimes he just wants cereal or toast so he usually gets a choice, otherwise you're just wasting what you're preparing. At dinner time he just has what he's given.

Children have much less control over the content of the main meal than over the other meals during the day and it is the one meal that the adults in the household consider it important for them to eat. Thus rejection of the meal as it is presented may not be rejection of the food but rejection of the control that is exercised through the provision and consumption of the food. In addition to this, the food that is provided at the main meal is, as we have already pointed out, usually in accordance with the father's wishes. This enforced consumption of the proper meal, therefore, also reinforces and symbolises the authority of the father within the family; it reinforces a patriarchal family structure. Acceptance of such a meal and conformity to it is ultimately an acceptance of the authority relations within the family; rejection of the meal or inappropriate behaviour at mealtimes can be an assertion of independence and an attempt to reject or modify the power and authority of a child's parents. Women are often aware of this: 'I think if you tell a kiddie "You eat it, it's good for you" then they won't. I know I never did. Oh cabbage, that's another one, greens are good for you, so I wouldn't eat cabbage for years. You do, you just rebel against it don't you?' Another woman told us:

Just because she got older, she knew her own mind, she got more fussy I suppose. I think it was just more that she was asserting herself as a person. If she said she wasn't going to eat it, then nobody could force her to – not that anybody did try to force her. I suppose she thought it was just a way of asserting herself when so much had to be done for her.

The scene is thereby set for the battle of wills over feeding which has now become a cliché of childcare advice literature. In this battle children possess only the negative sanctions of refusal and non-compliance, but these can be highly effective weapons. Women invest time and energy in the preparation of meals and children's refusal denies them the satisfaction and reward they may receive in seeing a meal consumed with relish and pleasure. This can prove very upsetting:

I used to get very uptight because if I'd cooked something I thought was nice and would do her a lot of good and she just wouldn't touch it. It's an emotional thing because apparently it's a sign of love when you cook. I hadn't really thought of it that way but I suppose it is. Because you feed your family that's one way of expressing love . . . and I realised I did get upset and of course she cottoned on – she's very bright – that was the way to really get me going.

Forcing children to eat food is not usually considered an appropriate response in these circumstances for this is distressing to women as well as children:

I only once lost my temper when Suzy was quite small, must have been over a year ago. And she'd asked me for something and hadn't eaten it and screamed and screamed. And I lost my temper and while she was screaming I dumped a spoonful in her mouth. And I was so appalled at what I'd done. There she was sitting there with food all over her face and screaming away.

The most common initial response is to take food away and hope that children will be ready to eat by the next mealtime, but if they continue to refuse meals they can effectively begin to exercise choice over the food that is provided. Parental authority, particularly mothers' authority, can in this way be challenged and eroded. Women frequently resort to giving children food they know they will like and eat rather than food which is considered better for them because food that is refused does no good at all and is also highly wasteful:

I'd rather give them something that I know they'll eat – there is absolutely no point in cooking something to throw it away. I used to feel I was giving them a good meal, for a long time even when I'd thrown it away I thought that at least I'd given them a good meal. It really did take a long time to get over this idea of a proper meal.

Children may be allowed to transgress the rules of socially acceptable eating behaviour if they provoke sufficient anxiety through their reluctance to eat food. Then children may be allowed to eat with their fingers rather than with implements:

I think being able to use a spoon and fork instead of their hands is important but I've given up on that one because she always uses her hands. She can do it, she used to do it. She can do it but for the moment it's gone by the board really. I'm so anxious she should put it in her mouth I don't really care how she does it.

In these desperate circumstances even the 'stealing' of food off others' plates may be permitted:

Actually, she does nick things off his [father's] plate, even when she wouldn't eat anything off her own plate. Normally I wouldn't agree with that – because he isn't keen – but like yesterday when she's not eating very much it's one way of getting her to eat.

Thus, by being firm in their refusal children may at least temporarily succeed in subverting the authority of their mothers over what they eat and how they eat it; the authority of the fathers, as we have seen, is another matter.

Despite the capitulation of women to their children's refusal of proper meals most of them still feel that their children *should* be eating them and are anxious about them if they do not. This concern arises because they feel that this is the only way of ensuring that they are eating 'properly' in terms of health as well as social acceptability. Indeed, they understand healthy eating as the regular consumption of food in the form of a proper meal. If children were eating a proper meal regularly then women assumed that they were eating healthily; healthy eating was interpreted within the social category of the proper meal. Conversely, if they were not eating proper meals then women became anxious about the child's diet and felt they were not eating properly, or were even not eating at all. One woman remarked on this elision: 'When I say not eaten I mean not eat meals – she'll have a packet of crisps you see or a piece of toast and she'll be quite happy with that sort of thing.' Children's eating habits, whether considered problematic or not, were almost always described in terms of their consumption of the main 'proper' meal of the day. Thus the faddiness, changeable likes and dislikes, varying appetite and preference for raw foods which characterised many children's eating all related to the main meal. Consumption of the other meals was not seen as having the same importance and between meals food consumption was often hardly classed as eating at all. Thus social eating in the form of consuming the proper meal with the rest of the family was the only form of eating which was considered to be proper for health reasons and for reasons of social conformity and adherence to accepted social practice. One woman, after filling in the diary for two weeks, said 'You tend to think she should eat a cooked meal, a hot meal, but when you look at what she's eaten over the day it's ... I've decided it's not that important.' This underlines the fact that eating patterns are not nutritional necessities but social constructions and that these social constructions normally colour the ways in which nutritional needs are understood. It was possible for children to be eating in a way that was nutritionally, but not socially, acceptable, and some of the women spoke about this distinction. One woman said of her daughter:

Well, she's not a problem either, I mean the problem is with me in that it annoys me when she doesn't eat what I've cooked. But she too is getting bigger and appears to be relatively healthy so she's obviously not severely malnourished. So any problem there is a behavioural problem rather than a real feeding problem because she doesn't eat at the right times and I'm getting strict about this now.

This tension between social and nutritional needs is something that emerges again and again in women's accounts of their children's eating habits, and the attempt to satisfy nutritional need within specific social forms gives rise to many of the problems mentioned.

Sweet foods as treats

Women feel they have to ensure their children are eating a diet which will allow them to grow and develop healthily, and ensuring that they eat proper meals is seen as a crucial part of this process. But there is another important feature of children's eating which was frequently referred to in our interviews and that is the consumption of sweets.

Sweets and sweet foods were regarded as part of the pleasure of childhood and women themselves enjoyed treating children with sweet foods. On the other hand, to ensure that children ate properly they often felt they had to restrict or at least *control* their child's consumption of sweet foods. This produced a contradictory situation and a conflict between giving a child food that is pleasurable to eat and ensuring that she/he eats food that is 'good for you'. Despite this contradiction almost all the women shared in the cultural assumption that children are entitled to sweets and that sweet giving and eating is an integral part of childhood. Almost half the women (87 – 44%) gave their children sweets on a daily basis, with social class I and II families less likely to do this than others (26% compared with 50%). Women who tried to ration their child's sweet intake, for whatever reason, felt that they were depriving them of one of the pleasures of childhood and felt guilty at their lack of generosity. This guilt came through in phrases such as, 'Aren't I awful?' and 'Don't I sound mean?' The comments of one woman who never gave her child sweets convey both the cultural expectation that children should receive sweets and the deprivation that may be implied in their denial: 'She has them at my mum's . . . they always have a lot of sweets there so she does have them. I don't think I could deprive her that much to make her different.' This points to the fact that women's control over their child's food intake was often undermined by other family members, most frequently the child's grandparents and father, and by people who were not closely involved with the child at all. We will look in some detail at the way these practices undermine women's control over the food intake of their children before going on to look at the other uses to which sweet foods are put within the mother-child relationship.

Children's assumed entitlement to sweets seems to override the rights as well as the responsibilities normally conferred on mothers to control their children's food consumption. One woman told us of the disrespect for her authority which was the way she interpreted a neighbour's assumption of rights, as far as sweet giving is concerned, over her children.

There's many a time when I've come out of the paper shop and they've been sat there with sweets in their hand. I think who's give them them. Round the corner you'll meet one of your neighbours who'll say 'I bought them you know'. It's good-hearted but in the wrong way . . . now I've learnt my lesson with other children and I say to their mothers 'Can they have?' and I'll whisper it before I'll let them hear, rather than upset them about it. I think you learn your lesson through having your own kids like that. You meet a lot of people who just thrust them into their hands and they think it's good. They give them a big bar of chocolate and things like that, that would last mine a couple or maybe three days but it can't be helped unfortunately.

And another woman forcefully expressed her resentment at being left so powerless.

Some people . . . are actually giving it to the child as they're saying, 'Can he have it?' Well I'm sorry but there's no way that I can not give it to him except snatch it out of his hand, which is a bit awkward because he might be having his lunch soon and I don't want him to have it, it's going to spoil lunch. But once he's got it in his hand there's not an awful lot I can do about it really except cause a scene, which isn't the kiddie's fault, it's the person that's giving it to James. They should ask me, not giving it to the child, you know, you can't really do much once they've got it in their hands really.

Visits between friends frequently occasion the use of sweets as gifts and often sweets and biscuits are offered to visiting children as a form of hospitality. Even if mothers themselves do not engage in these practices it is difficult to prevent children from eating sweets and biscuits if they are amongst friends who do so. Children are likely to get upset if they do not receive what they see other children consuming, and women are also highly aware that refusal of a gift is likely to create offence: 'Usually, if I go to other people and they say "Here's some sweets" there's nothing much you can do about it really. I don't like sort of offending people.'

Women's authority over their children's food consumption is also undermined within the family itself. Fathers and grandparents, in particular, are a source of food treats for children. Here the situation is rather more complicated, for these gifts are seen as an appropriate marker of a child's relationship with these significant family members. It is not uncommon for women to remark on such practices as a 'normal' part of grandparenthood or fatherhood. One woman, for example, said of her husband:

On a Friday when he comes home from work he always brings them a bar of chocolate or if we go out for a walk somewhere later on he'll buy them a bag of chips; that's a treat they like that. Or if we go to a fair he'll buy them a hot dog or a candy floss – *the normal things*. (Our emphasis.)

While another woman said of her parents: 'They give them sweets and crisps and chocolate like grandparents usually do.' Most women, however, experience tension between allowing grandparents and fathers to indulge children with sweets as a symbol of love and affection and maintaining their own control over children's eating. Grandparents may ally themselves with children against mothers' express wishes.

[Grandparents] give them sweets when I tell them not to. Because it's breaking all the rules. It takes about two days to get over going to see them on Sunday because everything that you've done during the week is just gone. One very fine example was about three weeks ago. Martin wouldn't eat his dinner so of course he was hungry in the afternoon and my mum said 'Can he have some chocolate?' and I said 'No'. She took them in the house and gave them chocolate. When they came out she said 'No, I haven't' but the evidence was there. But you don't like to push it too far because it upsets them.

Children may also ally with their fathers and capitalise on the differences which sometimes exist between parents in their attitudes to eating between meals.

He always says if they want it let them have it . . . You see with our Jan – I mean if he's at home working down there – 'Can I have a biscuit 'cos it's tea time?' 'Oh course you can have a biscuit.' But then it's 'Can I have another one, can I have another one' and Daddy sort of says 'Yes' you see and he says 'Well, let her eat when she wants to eat'. I say 'Yes but it's always the wrong things that you let her have!' . . . but more often than not it's me that's around to supervise what she's putting in.

Some women feel it is important to talk to their mothers about giving sweets to the children:

I have to tell my mum off a bit . . . I must tell her because otherwise if Gemma went there she'd probably get a packet a day which she's not used to. [Her mother says] 'Oh come on, children are allowed sweets', but I just don't think to a big extent they are . . . not if Gemma's prone to be on the big side anyway.

A common way of retaining control but at the same time accepting food gifts offered by grandparents is to ensure that they do not give sweets directly to their grandchildren: 'I think she's beginning to learn now. She used to be always bringing sweets down at half past eight in a morning but now she'll give me 'em and I'll dole 'em out.'

Interestingly, and significantly, such open questioning or control of men's practice is hardly ever attempted by women, although they often comment that their husbands are more likely to offer children food treats than they are themselves, and that fathers may be more indulgent generally towards eating between meals. In part, this attitude may be viewed as an appreciation that the giving of food treats plays an important role in emphasising a father's involvement with his children when he has to be away from them for long periods of time and is not very involved in their feeding and care. Sweet-giving by fathers often forms an important ritual in children's lives. This is particularly clear in the common practice of men bringing sweets home with them on a Friday evening after work, thus indicating the end of the working week and re-establishing the relationship between father and child: 'When he comes home on a Friday it's sort of a tradition that he brings them back something. It's usually a packet of sweets or a bar of chocolate – something which they wouldn't have under normal circumstances.' Some women certainly view their partner's treat-giving as a way of compensating children for their absence. 'He buys her sweets at the weekend. Probably 'cos he's not seen much of her during the week.' It is also interesting to note that men who are most involved with their children are least likely to give food treats. Only 58% of fathers who shared childcare when they were not at work outside the home give the children sweets as compared with over 70% of fathers who were less closely involved with their children.

The fact that men's treat-giving is rarely challenged by mothers may, however, also constitute a further instance in which women defer to the authority of their husband. This certainly appears clear when fathers are stricter about food treats than mothers, as was sometimes the case. One woman, for example, said of her own practice:

> Probably if I'd gone to the shop now I'd maybe have bought her a bag of crisps . . . if I buy a tube of Opal Fruits or gums she never gets the full tube in her hand. I break some off and spin it out for 2 or 3 days, y'know – as they definitely would put her off her meal – straight away my husband'd say 'What's she been having?' And he knows you see, and I'm in trouble again, so I'd better not.

Another woman reported that since her husband had started working from home he had become more aware of the number of sweets eaten by the children and did not approve: 'Now he's at home more he'll say "Are they having more sweets?" But then he hasn't had to look after them you know and I do sometimes think they're necessary – like if they've fallen.'

Such statements echo the feelings mothers express about the stricter attitudes fathers may have about children eating up meals. Fathers thus have the right to treat children and, apparently, they have the right to challenge mothers' own decisions about treating children. In so doing, they may be seen as exercising authority over women as well as children within the family.

Sweet foods, comfort and control

The last comment quoted above alerts us to the fact that the giving of sweets may be regarded by women as a necessary or unavoidable response to the problems presented by full-time childcare and it is to a more detailed consideration of this that we now turn. Women often find themselves using sweet food for many purposes other than the satisfaction of their children's hunger or even the simple practice of providing treats for children's pleasure.

Relatively isolated in the home with no-one to help carry the burden of caring, women find it difficult to maintain constant patience and inventiveness in their relations with their children. Children often nag for food when they are bored and they can be vociferous in their demand for sweets. This may be difficult for women to tolerate or ignore:

In the summer we don't have any problems at all because she's in and out through the back and she's quite happy. But when she's cooped up, she likes her freedom and she gets nattery . . . She wants more sweets when she's crabby 'Can I have a sweet?' or something, and I don't give in to her unless I absolutely have to. I try not to. Sometimes I give in, it depends, if I know that a sweet will keep her quiet and she'll be happy with one then perhaps I give in to her with one and then after that no more.

Children also demand constant attention and food may serve as a substitute for attention when women require some respite from keeping their children amused and occupied or children are being particularly obstreperous. Women do not view this practice very positively, but most feel driven to it on occasion:

Sweets are one of those awful things, you use sweets for such a lot of things and perhaps don't realise it at the time . . . to shut them up sometimes. I will admit to that. There have been times when I've just thought 'Oh, God, they'll have to shut up!' and I've given them something.

Childcare has to be combined with women's domestic tasks and other activities. Thus women find themselves using food as a means of quietening and occupying children in order to free themselves for the necessary labours of housework and meal preparation:

Usually I do it if I need to get on with something. It's amazing, they are all playing all nicely and then when you start a job, as soon as you start, they are both on top of you. Just 'cos you're doing something different they want to be in on it as well and they all want attention at the same time. So I find if I give them a biscuit or a dish of smarties or something it keeps them out of my way while I get on.

These sorts of occasions involve the use of food as a substitute for attention. Food may also more obviously represent comfort, as when sweets are used as a 'cure' for injuries:

I'm afraid I have fallen into the trap of having a magic sweetie to make it better. When they were little a magic rub would do, and then they would say 'It still hurts'. Then my magic wasn't very strong, so they do usually. If it's just a minor thing they don't get anything but Rebecca now says 'I need a sweet to make it better', but she does fall over a lot.

Children are also given food when they are fretful and sweets, in particular, are given to quieten and distract children who are distressed when their mothers temporarily leave them in the

care of others. Given the widespread nature of these practices it
is perhaps not surprising that we find food being used to
alleviate boredom and as a form of comfort by adults themselves. Interestingly, women have in the past seemed more
likely to view food in this way than men, but with increasing
male unemployment men seem also to be adopting these
practices. This suggests that it is partly the isolation and
boredom of the home which precipitates the use of food for these
purposes. That food may symbolise a mother's temporarily
withdrawn attention, and sometimes affection, is particularly
well portrayed by one woman who said:

I've been in a bad mood perhaps, and James hasn't had an awful lot of
attention or I maybe don't – he's just too much and mummy's not
feeling too bright either, you know, like the other day I didn't feel very
well, I thought 'Oh I've ignored him all day' I've just sort of gone
through the system you know of feeding him, changing him, putting
him to bed. Not really playing with him, just left him with the toys, you
know, so I think 'Oh well, pet, I'll give you some nice jelly, you like
jelly'.

Women sometimes only become aware that they are using
food in this manner when they reflect on the occasions upon
which children are given sweets, but food can also be used
in a more direct and conscious way to influence children's
behaviour. The fact that women control access to food means
that children can be denied those foods they covet most –
usually sweets – if they are not behaving well: 'Well I suppose on
occasions I have bribed Michael. Well, bribe is probably not the
right word, probably withheld is more the right word. If he's
doing something and I want him to stop I would probably say
"Well you don't get any sweets tomorrow".' Conversely, sweets
can be offered as a reward or incentive toward good behaviour.

If she's real good, I mean some days she's exceptionally good. She's very
good with him [younger brother], she's very sensible. I mean I can leave
him in here and I can go in there and I know that he won't touch the fire
or the television simply because she will shout before he gets anywhere
near, or she will get hold of him until I come back. If she's been real
helpful on a particular morning when I've been really busy I tend to say
'You can have some sweeties'.

If I have to take them to an aunt's or something like that and I want
them to behave themselves I usually sit them all in a row and give them

the pep talk before we set off. And I usually say 'Now if you behave yourselves, we'll have ice cream for tea, as a treat you see, or I'll take you to the sweet shop or you can have a lolly while you're out'.

Children might also be offered sweets or biscuits as a reward or an incentive for learning. This was particularly true in the case of potty training. Many women did not find these practices desirable – as one woman said 'It's a bit like Pavlov's dogs isn't it?' – but they were often found to be remarkably effective: 'I don't agree with it but I did reward her. I haven't done before but I did it with her. When she performed she was given a sweet and it worked amazingly. She was potty trained much quicker than the other two were.' Women who do not give their children sweets appreciate that they may thereby deny themselves a valuable bargaining aid in negotiations with their children.

I praise her, I wouldn't, I don't want to give her sweets – I haven't, not so far. I don't know whether I'm going to do so in the future because – when – I haven't got any lever at the moment to sort of, uhm, stop her any little privileges, do you know what I mean, so, uhm, I have to consider that. I could then withdraw something if she did something naughty.

It is also true to say, however, that if children receive sweets frequently as a matter of course their value as a reward or a comfort may be significantly diminished.

There are occasions when it is harder to resist the giving of food than others. The management of young children in public places is found to be especially problematic in this respect. The strategies which many women adopt in the home to distract or pacify their children when they are fretful or bad-tempered, such as reading stories, playing games and so on, are not usually suitable for the environment of a busy supermarket or a crowded bus or street. Bouts of crying or sulking and non-co-operation which might be ignored at home create embarrassment for women when they occur in a public place: 'If she does get upset in the shops I'll give her a biscuit then to keep her quiet. But if she was at home I wouldn't. If I'm out I can't stand her making a noise or seeing her red face.' Here we again see evidence that women's practices may be a response to significant social pressures. In describing their embarrassment women are aware of the fact that a child who is noisy or disruptive may be taken as evidence of their own inadequacies as mothers. In the same way children who are messy in their eating habits or who do not eat proper meals are a 'bad' reflection of their mother's child-rearing practices. Women thus find themselves using food as a means of controlling children's behaviour and this may frequently conflict with their desire to control food consumption itself. Even women who are very strict about not letting their children eat between meals appreciate the difficulties of these sorts of situations.

I can see the temptation. I mean I'm not so detached from the rest of the world that I can't obviously. I think I would be mad myself simply giving him a biscuit because . . . but supposing I was waiting for a bus somewhere and he was screaming his head off and I had in my pocket a plain biscuit I would give it to him to shut him up.

All these practices, therefore, may be viewed as representing women's response to the frequently problematic business of childcare in our culture. They also show the way in which sweet foods can be used by women to *control* a child's behaviour, to stop them crying, to distract them, even to potty train them. Sweet foods are used to manipulate, if that is not too strong a word, children's behaviour.

It is interesting that food used in this way is never part of a proper meal. Indeed, sweet foods are often not viewed as food at all, they are 'goodies' and treats, the inessentials of a child's diet which perform functions other than ensuring health and development. It seems that the non-essential character of sweet food is what lends itself to being used as a reward or a comfort, a bribe or a treat. Food that constitutes the proper meal is regarded as essential for a child's health and is therefore simply not available to be used in this way.

A few women, a minority who were mainly middle class, made a conscious effort not to use food in this way. This was usually because they did not want their child to learn to associate food with comfort: ' . . . last week you asked me if we'd had any dietary touble in the family. I thought afterwards, two of us have had anorexia, and I'm trying to avoid her getting the type of likeness for food that I used to have, y'know, seeing it as a comfort.' However, this type of awareness was not widespread and in most families children were being taught that food is a comfort and compensation, something to turn to when you are bored or upset. Children learn through these practices that food not only satisfies hunger but that it satisfies all sorts of other emotional needs as well. They also learn, through their adaptation to and acceptance of the proper meal, about relations of power and domination according to gender and age within the family.

Age differences in food consumption

These gender and age relations are also manifest in the way food is distributed *between* family members, and we wish to explore this in some detail. Table 5.1 presents women's, men's and children's frequency of consumption of certain food items over a two-week period. This was again taken from the women's diary records.

As we have already noted (Chapter 4), foods are ranked in a hierarchy, and have different social values attached to them. In addition, certain foods, often of relatively low social status, are regarded as 'children's' food within British culture. This is true of sweets, crisps, fish fingers, baked beans, 'noodle doodles', breakfast cereal and so on. These types of food are marketed as being particularly suitable for children and it is children who are depicted eating them in advertising campaigns. They are made for 'little mouths' and 'little fingers', or so the slogans tell us. These foods are, by and large, regarded as low social status, perhaps reflecting their association with children. Indeed, they are consumed more frequently by children than adults which, we would argue, reflects children's lesser status in comparison to adults within the family. As we can see in Table 5.1, there are certain foods which are eaten more frequently by children than by adults. These are low status fish (e.g., fish fingers), fresh fruit, breakfast cereal, biscuits, puddings, sweets, soft drinks, crisps, foods like baked beans, tinned spaghetti, etc., and milk. They are all foods which are generally associated with children, either because they are thought to be good for them, as with milk and fresh fruit, or because children particularly like them for the reasons we have elaborated above. The foods that enjoy a high social status, particularly meat, cake and alcohol, are however eaten more frequently by adults than children, and this we would argue is a reflection and marker of power and status divisions within the family. Vegetables, the component of the proper meal which children were most often reported as disliking, were eaten less frequently by them than by adults,

Table 5.1 *Average incidence of consumption of all food items over a 2-week period*

	Women	Men	Children
High status meat	4·5	4·9	3·1
Medium status meat	6·8	9·0	5·3
Low status meat	5·1	6·8	5·2
Whole fish	1·7	1·9	0·9
Low status fish	1·6	1·5	1·7
Eggs	4·4	5·1	3·5
Cheese	5·6	5·8	3·8
Green leafy vegetables (cooked)	2·9	2·8	2·1
Other vegetables (cooked)	7·9	8·2	6·8
Raw vegetables	5·0	5·3	2·3
Fresh fruit	5·9	5·2	7·3
Potatoes (boiled/roast)	6·4	6·6	6·3
Chips	7·0	7·0	4·0
Bread	19·0	21·6	17·4
Pasta/rice	1·1	1·2	0·7
Breakfast cereal	5·2	5·3	10·4
Cakes	6·7	7·3	4·9
Biscuits	8·0	6·4	11·3
Puddings	7·0	7·0	9·3
Sweets	3·5	2·6	8·1
Soft drinks	2·7	2·0	22·5
Crisps	1·8	2·4	4·0
Baked beans, etc.	1·9	2·0	2·9
Pulses/nuts	0·2	0·1	0·2
Soup	1·5	1·0	1·3
Milk	6·0	6·3	21·5
Cream	0·8	0·9	0·5
Tea/coffee	58·0	54·3	13·4
Alcohol	2·7	4·4	0·2

as were potatoes (slightly) and meat, particularly high and medium status meat. This may reflect the difficulties that women experience in getting children to eat proper meals, but it also reflects many women's views that it would be a waste to give children the best steak, which they would not appreciate. This type of meat was often difficult for children to chew and it was hard for them to cope with the cutting up necessary to get the food to their mouths. It is also a meat of high social status, and higher frequency of consumption of this high status meat can be understood as reflecting the social status of the consumer. Thus in these terms alone it is not appropriate for children to eat it.

The frequency of cake and alcohol consumption, which are also endowed with a high social status, is much lower for children than for adults, and whereas tea and coffee are drunk by adults, soft drinks or milk are given to children. Hardly any children were given tea or coffee; they were felt to be too strong for them, although some young children might be given weak tea on occasions. Children were hardly *ever* given alcoholic drink apart from the odd sip of sherry or shandy from their parents' or grandparents' glass.

My nana is still alive, she's nearly 90, and she normally comes for two holidays a year, she's one of those people that believes in having a glass of sherry every day. She brings it with her when she comes, and of course when she gets her glass out to have a drink our two normally get their glasses out, but that's the only time that they have a drink of any sort really. She gives them a little, tiny drop in the bottom, and they both like that when she has one you see.

In one or two families where wine was a more frequent occurrence, children might drink it very much watered down. But this was confined to a very few of the more middle-class families. 'If we have wine, I'll let her have a bit, I usually dilute it. I know I perhaps shouldn't let her have it but my opinion is that if they come to respect things like that they're not going to go overboard with it.'

It is interesting to look at differences in frequency of consumption of certain low status and high status foods amongst children of different ages. As with changes in birthday food, it seems that food consumed on a daily basis marks the stages of a child's advance towards adult status. In Table 5.2 we can see the frequency of consumption of 'children's' food according to age; most of these foods have a relatively low social value attached to them.

It is clear from this Table that consumption of foods in Group 1 is highest for the lowest age groups and decreases most sharply after the age of 5, when children start school. Consumption of

Table 5.2 *Age variations in frequency of consumption of 'children's' foods over a two-week period. (Low status meat is included here as, although children do not consume it more often than men, they do consume it more often than women)*

	0–2 yrs (n = 126)	3–5 yrs (n = 108)	6–11 yrs (n = 50)
(Group 1)			
Milk	24·6	20·1	15·8
Puddings	10·3	9·1	7·8
Squash/soft drinks	24·4	24·5	15·6
Breakfast cereal	10·9	10·3	9·2
Biscuits	11·3	11·6	10·4
Fresh fruit	7·2	7·4	6·9
Baked beans, etc.	3·2	2·8	2·8
(Group 2)			
Sweets	7·3	9·0	8·6
Crisps	2·6	4·4	6·7
Low status meat	4·7	5·8	6·0
Low status fish	1·5	1·9	1·7

most of the foods also shows a decrease between the 0 – 2 year age group and the 3 – 5 year age group. This is particularly clear for milk, puddings and breakfast cereal, foods which are felt to be important for young children. Several of the women commented on the importance of breakfast and milky puddings for young children. On the other hand, sweet and crisp consumption seems to increase with increasing age, perhaps reflecting the increasing ability of children to determine their own food intake and their inclusion in 'pack-ups' that children take to school. The foods mentioned so far are usually regarded as 'children's' food, but the frequency of consumption of more 'adult' food also varies with age; this is shown in Table 5.3. As we can see, the consumption of medium and low status meat, cakes, raw vegetables and chips tends to increase with age, reflecting changing eating patterns as children grow older. Foods of high status, however, such as high status meat and alcohol, do not reflect differences in age between children although they are consumed considerably less frequently by children of all ages than by adults.

It seems then that the distribution and consumption of food, as well as reflecting gender status within families, reflect age

Table 5.3 *Variation in frequency of consumption of certain foods by age of child*

	0 – 2 yrs (n = 126)	3–5 yrs (n = 108)	6–11 yrs (n = 50)
High status meat	2·7	3·6	3·1
Cakes	3·8	5·3	6·7
Alcohol	0·1	0·3	0·2
Tea/coffee	10·8	14·7	18·0
Chips	3·4	4·5	4·3
Medium status meat	4·8	5·6	6·2
Low status meat	4·7	5·8	6·0
Green cooked veg	2·1	2·0	2·1
Other cooked veg	6·7	6·8	6·6
Bread	16·0	18·8	18·0
Potatoes	6·3	6·5	6·1
Raw vegetables	1·7	2·4	3·3

status, most clearly between adults and children but also between children of different ages. The food eaten every day at home, therefore, marks social status and reflects social relations and divisions within families.

Children's food needs

Differential distribution of food in this way is justified and explained with reference to food 'needs', a seemingly biologically determined and natural phenomenon. Supposed differences in food needs between men and women, as we have already seen, are justified and explained by reference to men's work being more physically strenuous than women's (even when they are in a sedentary occupation), men being bigger than women and by virtue of that fact alone needing more food, and, simply, the unquestioned assumption that men always eat more than women – don't they? It is difficult in the case of adult-child divisions in food consumption to disentangle cultural assumptions from physiologically based arguments and the power exercised by children themselves over their own food intake. We have already indicated that within British culture there are certain expectations that children's food needs will be different from those of adults. Milk, cereal and fresh fruit are thought to be important for children's growth. This view is backed up by health care professionals and food distribution within families indicates that these views are borne out by practice. In addition to this, there is also the culture of childhood which deems childhood to be a time free from responsibility, of pleasure without a thought for the future. Treating children with sweet foods and indulging them with food that they enjoy eating is part of this, and again the data on food consumption bears this out. Children do, indeed, consume more sweets, biscuits, puddings and crisps than do adults. There are also foods which are not felt to be appropriate for children, and these seem to have little scientific basis being culturally specific. In this category come the views commonly held by women, that children cannot manage raw vegetables, in the form of salads for instance, that tea and coffee are not good for them, that strong, spicy foods will upset children's tummies, and that alcohol is an adult's drink. This latter prohibition is backed by law and by medical opinion. Children are clearly regarded as different from adults in terms of the food which is appropriate for them. They have to learn to eat properly, to eat proper meals as other members of the family, but their full assumption of adult eating patterns only occurs gradually and is a process fraught with potential conflict.

The women's accounts of feeding children reveal not only that age influences the way children are fed but also gender. Our quantitative data, as we have already indicated, show that the frequency of meat consumption is higher among boys than girls. The figures for other foods are not so conclusive, but women's views on gender differences between children are significant. In quantitative terms, few of the women, when asked directly, thought there was any difference between the food needs of boys and girls. In fact, only 4 (2%) thought there were gender based differences among pre-school age children, while 181 (90·5%) thought there were not. However, despite these responses many of the women's comments reveal that they did differentiate on the basis of gender. Their differing views and expectations of children's eating requirements often mirrored the distinctions they made between men's and women's food needs. Boys were said to need more food than girls because they were bigger or because they expended more energy. The comments below illustrate these points:

I think people make them different. I've got a friend who's got two boys and they treat them differently. They definitely eat more. But they're meant to eat a bit more aren't they? Because they're meant to be slightly heavier – in the book I've got – the whole way through. So there must be something there – but maybe it's just they're bigger.

Fathers play with their boys a lot more so they must use a lot more energy and get a lot hungrier, whereas you don't rough little girls about.

Even when it appeared that women did not think there were any gender-based differences between young children their later explanations revealed that they were making these sorts of distinctions:

I think they might develop different things as they get older but I can't see that young children will just have different tastes just because they are one or the other sex. [Do you think they probably have the same food needs?] Well again I think it depends on the kids. I think probably kids do rush around a lot and use a lot of energy which maybe boys do more than girls, and so maybe they need more.

Even at this early age girls' 'femininity' could be invoked as something that would lead to their eating less than boys, a precursor of the emphasis on dieting and slimness that becomes much more apparent with the onset of puberty: 'I think boys are probably a bit more adventurous, a bit quicker, I don't know, but little girls are daintier – they tend to eat less usually, but you know not having a little girl you can't really say.' It is interesting, in the light of our findings that women consume biscuits and sweets more frequently than men, that some women felt that girls showed a preference for sweet foods in a way that boys did not. Their views echo the nursery adage that girls are made of 'sugar and spice and all things nice' in contrast to boys who originate from 'slugs and snails and puppy dogs' tails.' One woman said: 'I think boys are more keen on savouries while girls like sweet things.' And another voiced similar views:

I think boys like different sorts of textures to girls. They might prefer the rougher types of things like beefburgers, whereas girls might relish ice cream, strawberries and cream, y'know, softer things – but maybe that's me psychologically thinking they're tougher. I picture boys eating more rougher things and girls eating – well sugar and spice and all things nice.

One woman told us of her experience during pregnancy:

I'd say Darren's taken to more savoury things, he won't eat cake, and I'd say Tracy is more on the sweet side ... I don't know if it's a coincidence, but when I was pregnant with Darren I ate more savoury things and when I was having Tracy it was more sweet things.

These opinions reveal that although most women, when asked directly about gender differences in the food needs of pre-school age children, said that they did not think there was any difference, many of them subscribed to a gender-based ideology of food needs even among very young children. Indeed, our quantitative data supports the existence of gender-based feeding practices, particularly in the case of meat which is, arguably, the most gender-sensitive food in the British diet. However, it is true to say that the gender divisions in frequency of food consumption were less marked among pre-school age children than among older children and adults, and we would link this difference to the asexuality that is ascribed to young children within British culture. Many more women believe that food needs are different for male and female children once puberty is reached. This is significant because it clearly links food consumption to ideologies of sexuality. Certain patterns of food consumption are considered appropriate for women while others are appropriate for men, and these consumption patterns are aimed at achieving the 'ideal' body size and body image which is smaller for women than for men. As children grow older it is expected that they will adopt the eating patterns appropriate to their sex; this became very clear from our discussions with the women themselves.

We asked the women whether they thought that children's food needs changed as they grew older and their replies indicated that gender is very important in shaping attitudes towards food needs, particularly when children begin to mature sexually. Of the women 90 (45%) thought that boys' and girls' food needs changed as they got older, either because of boys' greater physical activity or girls' consciousness of their weight, or both, while 53 (26·5%) thought there was no divergence in food needs. The other women either did not know (21) or definitely thought there was no gender specificity in food needs (19 – 9·5%). In the women's comments we again find reference to the 'fact' that boys tend to be more active and therefore use up more energy and need more food than girls. Also women commonly mentioned that girls began to be figure-conscious as they reached their teens and this reduced the amount they ate. Some typical comments are presented below:

When they get older I think boys need more filling up. When they get to 9 or 10 they seem to be eating twice as much – you probably have to fill them up with more potatoes and bread. [Why?] Well I think they've got more natural energy. Maybe it's just mine . . . but these two [boys] seem to have more energy than Gemma.

They'll probably change their habits of food when they get older. Probably get more fussy. [When they're teenagers?] Oh well they did in my house – and girls get onto slimming.

Even those few women who insisted that there was no difference in food needs between the sexes unconsciously slipped into the assumption that if there were a difference it would be that girls ate less than boys; a clear indication of the power of this ideology.

One woman emphatically denied any differences in food needs:

No again – I mean I eat the same things as my husband and we're different sexes. No I think – Crikey! – I don't know why you've got that question down there really. [Well some people think there's a difference.] Well, blimey, I mean we're made the same way. There's nothing different about us as far as food is concerned so why should we eat different? I don't see why girls should eat smaller portions than boys unless they want to but I don't think you can generalise about that can you?

She was, however, unusual. Most women felt that there were clear gender-based differences, if not in actual physiological *needs*, at least in food habits. These differences became apparent as children grew into young adults and adopted the different cultural trappings of masculinity and femininity, the masculine image being one of activity and large body size, the feminine image in contrast being one of slightness in body, relative inactivity and low expenditure of energy.

Clearly, then, feeding children is not only a process of meeting physiological need, although this seems to be the way it is understood, particularly by health care professionals. Within the dominant ideology it is naturalised and understood as meeting needs that are, in some way, biologically determined.

Clearly there *is* a physiological need for food, it would be absurd to claim otherwise. But the way this need is met and the cultural forms within which it is satisfied are socially constructed and determined. Feeding children, which is primarily a woman's task, therefore not only ensures that a child grows and develops, but also teaches them about social divisions within the family, relations of power and subordination, and that food has a myriad of social meanings and functions other than that of alleviating hunger. Women, in teaching children socially acceptable eating habits, in comforting children with food, and in demonstrating by the way food is distributed between father, mother and children, social divisions and relations, are initiating children into the social order. And children's eventual acceptance of all the rules and proprieties governing eating, particularly those surrounding the proper meal, is an acceptance and naturalisation of the social divisions which characterise the patriarchal family within British society.

6

Women, health and diet

A change in eating habits has become increasingly prominent amongst the suggested contributions people may make to an improvement in health and well-being. The fashionable status of nutritional concerns is evidenced by a plethora of recent books on how to achieve a healthy diet and the frequent parading of food 'experts' in the mass media more generally. In this chapter we explore women's views on the relation between food and health and the impact of these views on their own and their families' diets. We will show that although almost all women feel that food is important to health, quoting phrases such as 'You are what you eat', when pressed they find it very hard to elaborate the connections. They agree with the general idea that food must bear some relation to health, but what exactly this relation is remains vague and uncertain. Similarly women's knowledge of nutrition remains uneven and confused. In spite of this vagueness women were very concerned that the family should eat properly and, as we have already pointed out, worried or felt guilty if their children or their partners went without a proper meal. If this happened then they were not eating 'properly'. In fact, most women assessed the nutritional value of food through this social category. However, women did hold views on the goodness of food, whether it was fattening or not, whether certain foods filled you up without doing you any good. These categories and classifications can be understood as women's conceptions of the healthiness, or otherwise, of food and as such provide an important means of uncovering social definitions of the relation between food and health. These social definitions and understandings often inform women's practices in ways which nutritional and supposedly scientific principles do not. Indeed, women's views on 'expert' opinion are often marked by a (healthy) scepticism. Thus although women appear to be vague on the specific links between food and health, their attitudes and practices reveal that *social* definitions of the relation between food and health often affect a family's diet.

The women were asked whether the food we eat is important for our health and almost all of them said that it was. In fact only 2 out of the 200 women said it was not important, and 5 others were unsure whether there was any link. At the most basic level, women felt food was important to keep you going, it was the fuel that the body needed: 'Well you wouldn't put cheap fuel in a car and if you want your body to keep going for a hundred years you shouldn't put rubbish in it.' This view was widespread and many women commented that they needed to eat properly in order to cope with the demands placed on them by children, husbands and housework. If they did not eat properly they felt tired, weak and irritable.

If you don't eat properly . . . if you don't eat a proper meal you can get yourself run down and that. If you're working I think you sort of need it for energy. 'Cos I know, like for example, if I've not eaten before I've gone to work, when I'm there I'm feeling right . . . more or less like flaking out and sort of if you've had a meal you can keep going better.

Good food was frequently cited as being the key factor in healthy growth and development or, as it was most commonly referred to, 'Healthy teeth and bones'. In addition women mentioned the benefit of a good diet in keeping skin clear and hair shiny; here we are reminded of the advice commonly meted out in women's magazines. Good food was also thought to have value in making your nails strong, warding off colds and helping to prevent illness generally, it helps people's recovery from illness and 'keeps you regular'. Poor diet was implicated in obesity, tooth decay, hair in poor condition, spots and constipation, and specific illnesses such as bowel disease and heart disease. However, most women assumed that their family's diet was healthy unless they actually suffered from ill health, such as continuous colds during the winter or bowel problems. Thus health was defined as the absence of illness: 'We haven't much illness, none of us hardly ever go to the doctor and I'm sure it must be what we eat because it's the kind of staple of life, isn't it, food?' But the shakiness of the belief in a close link between food and health is brought out by women's observations of people who, in their opinion, do not eat a proper diet but still appear to be healthy: 'I mean there's a kid down the street who eats chip sandwiches all the time and they don't get any illnesses whatsoever. I mean they can live like crows can kids and still survive and yet I worry and fret about making sure he gets the right things.' And for many women it was almost an act of faith to believe that such a link existed. The following comments illustrate this:

Well I'm sure it *must* affect how healthy you are, whether you're eating food that is nutritious. You don't see any strong evidence of this but I'm sure there must be. People on the most appalling diets seem quite healthy – I don't have any proof. I just feel it *must* have some effect.

Concern over children's diets and a belief in the importance of proper eating for them was, despite the reservations voiced by some women, widespread. However, women's own diets were not invested with nearly so much importance:

I don't really think of it for myself but I think you do when you've got children, you think about it. I mean I tend to think I eat what I like, you know, I don't think an awful lot about sort of health wise because I'm fairly fit, but with children I think you do – it's nice to know they've got some reserve you know, that the food they have had has done them some good.

Indeed, in the effort to ensure that children were properly fed women often did without. For instance at breakfast, a meal regarded as important for children, women were usually so busy organising everyone for work and school that their own needs for food went unmet. The problems and tensions of feeding children often led women to neglect themselves, either by going without food or by finishing off whatever the children had failed to eat. Given this maternal self sacrifice it is perhaps not surprising that women commented on feeling run down and linked this with their own diets. But together with this self-neglect women shoulder the main responsibility for ensuring the 'healthiness' of their families' diets. This is a respons-ibility that they feel and that professional health care advice emphasises; women are regarded as the guardians of their own and their families' health and providing a 'proper' diet is a basic element of this role. Women accept this, but it can lead to an increased burden of guilt if, for whatever reason, men and children cannot be provided with what women feel is a 'proper' diet. Women were conscious that responsibility for the family's health was part of being a wife and mother, and it could be a burden.

I didn't have so much time to worry about it when we were first married and when I was single, it was just there in me, I used to think 'I must read up on it or I must buy more health foods and things'. But now I'm at home all day and it's my job really to make sure everybody eats, well I class it as part of my job that everybody eats the right sort of thing, enough of everything, I read about it more – I worry about it more.

This general concern and feeling of responsibility towards the family's health did not mean that nutritional principles were at the forefront in determining the food a family ate. Women continuously *worried* about the 'goodness' of the diet, but this worry was translated into practice through the notion of eating 'properly'. Therefore as long as she provided the family with proper meals on a regular basis she felt their health needs were met. The family diet was therefore not constructed around principles of nutritional 'science', but around a social category which defined a diet which was regarded as socially *and* nutritionally adequate.

Having said this there were occasions when health concerns directly affected families' diets. This was usually where there had been an illness in the family in which diet had been implicated, or when a change of diet had been recommended by a medical practitioner. Two families, for example, ate a radically altered diet on the recommendation of a naturopath who had initially been consulted because of ill health. One of these women described the change.

I think it was two things really; one was when I had my hip operated on, which was just before I met Michael [husband]. I was advised to go and see this naturopath/osteopath because he would be able to help me with my joints. I went to him with that aim and he is a vegetarian and encourages vegetarian and wholefood diet and I listened to all of that and regarded it as cranky but I valued the other things he had to say. Michael went to see him as well because of Michael's own digestive problems the doctor suggested that more of a vegetarian diet would help him. Michael was also very sceptical about it but the seed was planted in a way and then shortly after that I suppose the wholefood revolution started to get hold of the press and so forth so he didn't appear to be simply a quack but, you know, sustained by other people's views. So there were two things going and then thirdly the wholefood bakery opened, which we pass every day and, little by little, the whole thing became unavoidable and we also recognised that we were actually much, much healthier as a result.

In the other family the woman's experience of colitis and severe migraine had similarly led to specialist consultation then a change in diet.

While few families had adopted a vegetarian or entirely wholefood diet, some other women had made certain adjustments to the existing diet. Allergies in children led to the avoidance of certain foods for the children concerned, e.g. dairy products or foods containing certain additives. The incidence of heart disease in the family sometimes led to avoidance of foods with a high fat content while bowel disease had often triggered a move towards more fibre in the diet. In general, it was clear that the rethinking of diet in this way was closely allied to the existence of illness. As one woman said, when pondering the changes made in her own family's diet because of the existence of allergy in the family, 'I think unless it affects you, you just don't bother'. Other women also commented on their own approaches to health and diet:

I eat wholemeal bread because my father-in-law died of cancer of the bowel actually and this is why I tend to be for roughage whereas I previously wasn't in the least bit interested. But you do become aware of those things through circumstances or something and so therefore something like that brings it home to you and you tend to think about it whereas, I mean if you don't know anybody who's had anything like that you just carry on in your own sweet way.

The importance of personal observation and experience is clear from these examples. Just as the appearance of health assures women that they are providing an adequate diet, the presence of illness close to home can convince them of the need to change their diets. In this way health concerns can become central to a family's diet.

However, for most of the women, these concerns remained peripheral and the family's diet was dependent on other social and cultural considerations. It was generally assumed that 'variety' and 'everything in moderation' guaranteed the 'goodness' of the diet. A typical comment was: 'I think if you have a varied diet and you eat different things, well, you're getting what you need out of most things aren't you?'

Nutritional knowledge

As we have already indicated, women's nutritional knowledge was often vague and confused. Many of them reported receiving advice to eat properly or to eat a balanced diet during pregnancy. But although they were all able to define proper eating in social terms, defining a balanced diet was much more problematic, and their health care advisers had apparently not thought to explain the terms. Almost a third of the women we spoke to hazarded that a balanced diet was 'a bit of everything': 'An everyday diet. Not cutting down on one thing and piling up on another. Just eating everything. Like people cut out bread and potato – a balanced diet is just a bit of everything in moderation.' Indeed, balanced meals seemed to be similar in composition to the proper meal; once again nutritional ideas are interpreted and understood within social categories. Few women talked of a balanced diet in terms of nutrients, and even among those that did their knowledge remained partial. It was far more common for women to mention certain foodstuffs as being essential for a balanced diet. Vegetables and meat were most frequently mentioned followed by fruit and dairy products (especially milk). Eggs, fish and cereals were mentioned by fewer women and hardly any (6) mentioned sugar or sweet foods. The way a balanced diet is understood and the importance of social categories and practices to the interpretation of this nutritional idea is brought out by the following comment

As I say, . . . I think he ate toast for his breakfast, sandwiches for his dinner, sandwiches for his tea, and although he's getting something in the sandwiches, salad and meat, it was bread three times you see and to me that was wrong. But it was just a hot day and he was so busy so that's what he wanted. No way would that be a balanced diet. I think you need a cooked meal every day really.

Similarly convenience foods could not provide a balanced diet, and again this underlines the way the idea of a 'proper' diet structures women's views on food and health.

I do think you need balanced food. It wouldn't be any good to eat frozen beefburgers and frozen peas every day and junk food all the time. I don't think it would do you any good, I think you would suffer from malnutrition eating the wrong things. If I gave Michele say for breakfast a slice of toast with jam on 'cos she'd eat it, and then for dinner frozen beefburgers and chips every day – give her a lot of junk – I don't think it would do her any good . . . I do think it's important to eat a good meal.

Given the interpretation and understanding of nutritional concepts through social categories, it is interesting to look at women's views on 'expert' nutritional opinion. Most women were very aware of the conflicting opinions over food and its effects on health that are expressed by the 'experts', and these contradictions and frequent changes in nutritional thinking led many women to take up a sceptical position on these issues. Again the centrality of the tried and tested proper meal is apparent. Listening to expert opinion can lead to the conclusion that almost *any*thing is bad for you: because of this most women adopt a strategy of sticking to the diet they have always eaten:

They throw that many things at you – this is not good for you, that is not good for you. I mean there's supposed to be a lot of fat in milk now isn't there? I mean at one time it was eat milk, eat cheese and eggs and butter and you'll be OK but they've found that with every one of these foods that they think there's something in that you shouldn't be eating so, no, I don't worry because we just wouldn't eat anything. We didn't have all this years ago, did we? All this, this is good for you, that's good for you, don't eat this, don't eat that and junk foods. I mean who thought of the word junk foods anyway? No, as I say, if I sat down and really thought about most of the things we ate, what I'd read about or what I'd seen on television, we wouldn't eat anything at all and we'd die from not eating, but at least I'd know from what we died.

It is not uncommon for women to say that greater knowledge of the potential dangers of the food they eat has increased their feelings of insecurity rather than helping them to make realistic decisions about diet. Cynicism is as likely to be expressed by those who read widely as by those whose contact with expert opinion is confined to the odd television or radio programme. One woman, who had herself been involved in health education, commented:

You see in the paper that – oh, you know – that you shouldn't eat Flora any more 'cos it gives you cancer of somewhere so you've got to go back to butter and then all the advertising comes about butter, but I mean if you actually read the BMJ [British Medical Journal] there's three articles saying it's a load of rubbish and, you know, it's all fashion really isn't it?

Women respond to these contradictions and changes in nutritional fashions by taking little notice of what the experts say. They stick to the diet that they have always known which is structured around the proper meal and contains a variety of different foods:

I've found the old traditional foods that we were told were good for us and then we went into the health food era where all the things we'd been told were good for you like porridge, bread, potatoes, was suddenly bad for you and now it's switched back again. The modern thinking now is that porridge is very good for you, potatoes and bread and things like that so I think it's gone full circle and I never listen to the experts . . . I think a little bit of everything and hopefully it'll balance out.

We would suggest that this type of reaction is not at all unreasonable or irrational in the face of constant changes in nutritional thinking. Indeed, when we were interviewing, dietary fibre was beginning to be pushed and the NACNE report was about to be published. This report heralded a significant shift in nutritional thinking. Where once the emphasis was placed on protein and vitamins, developments in nutritional theory have introduced more complex, and sometimes contradictory, concepts. The latest recommendations now emphasise the importance of reducing fats, sugar and salt and of increasing fibre in the diet (NACNE, 1983). This means that foods such as meat and dairy products which seemed to receive unreserved backing as good and valuable foods in the past are subject to criticism because of their high fat content, while foods such as bread and potatoes which have acquired the status of fattening 'fillers' in many people's minds are now promoted as useful sources of dietary fibre.

Most women seem to subscribe to the former emphasis placed on protein, in the form of meat, fish, cheese and eggs, and vitamins. These are the nutritional ideas they grew up with and protein and vitamins are often the only nutritional concepts they employ. Women commonly report being taught about the importance of protein and vitamins in their domestic science lessons at school and for many this provides the basis of any nutritional theory they may possess, although their memories of such teaching are characteristically vague: 'It started you off with basics and you still know which food contains proteins and which are the right kinds of food. It's still at the back of your mind even if you can't make a list of all the things you learnt.' Almost all women were taught domestic science at school but women in social classes I and II who generally went on to higher education were less likely to have received such teaching: 78% of women in social classes I and II took domestic science as compared with 96% in social class IIIN and all women in social classes IIIM, IV and V.

Most recent innovations in nutritional theory, most obviously the increasing importance attached to fibre in the diet, still seemed a long way from gaining acceptance with the majority of the women we spoke to. There were, however, significant class differences in awareness of these innovations and in practices relating to them and here women's own class was a more sensitive indicator of these attitudes and practices than that of their partners. For instance, women who were or had been in professional occupations were less likely to place stress on the importance of meat in the diet and more likely to express a desire to move towards a wholefood diet and increased consumption of fibre. An awareness of developments in nutritional thinking and its translation into practice, and the avoidance of sugar in beverages, was more commonly displayed by these women, as the following figures indicate. In classes I and II 48% of the women bought wholemeal bread compared with 13% of women in class IIIN, 10% of women in class IIIM and 6% of women in classes IV and V. No one had sugar in drinks in 57% of the families of women in classes I and II but this was true of only 14% of the families of women in classes IIIN and IIIM and 6% of the families of women in classes IV and V. This seems to indicate that new patterns of eating percolate through society gradually, beginning with those in the highest (in terms of the occupational hierarchy) social groups. It would appear, then, that the common image of vegetarianism and the consumption of wholefood as something indulged in by the middle class is not inaccurate. Strict vegetarianism was rare amongst the women we talked to, but all the families who forswore meat were middle class and it is women in the professions who generally patronise wholefood shops. Of women in social classes I and II 31% used wholefood shops as compared with 3% of women in classes IIIN and IIIM and no women in classes IV and V. In fact the class nature of an interest in wholefoods was brought out by several working-class women who felt very reluctant to go into the local wholefood shop. They did not feel comfortable there and preferred to shop at other more 'ordinary' shops, even though this meant they could not buy the more healthy foods that they would have preferred.

Middle-class women also seemed to be more informed and concerned about recent debates concerning the potential dangers to health in dietary practice. They were most likely to mention issues such as the link between cholesterol and heart disease, cancer and food additives, and hyperactivity as a form of food allergy. When they were specifically asked whether there was anything which they had heard recently about food or aspects of diet which worried them, 55% of I/II women mentioned cholesterol as compared with 30% of women in classes IIIN and IIIM and 28% of women in classes IV and V. The links between cancer and diet were a concern for 21% in classes I and II, 12% in IIIN, 10% in IIIM and 17% in IV and V. Hyperactivity was mentioned by 17% of women in classes I and II but by only two women in other social classes. They were also more likely to have made changes in their families' diets in response to information about dietary dangers or benefits. Of the women in occupational classes I and II 60% reported changing their food habits in response to information about food dangers, compared with 36% of the women in class IIIN, 41% of the women in class IIIM and 22% in classes IV and V. A fairly typical change was described by a teacher:

I think that what I think I should do is certainly move quite drastically towards a wholefood diet. I mean at the moment we have some notional interest in it in that we eat brown bread and we eat brown rice in an effort to cut out a lot of the additives, but it's done in a very mild way because there are other factors which infringe upon it. I think it's something that also comes in phases and like if I'm feeling miserable for any reason then I just don't care what we're eating. I think it's the time when you are feeling very much in control of situations that you have the luxury to work at something that might be regarded as a faddy diet. I think on the whole that we eat reasonably well.

Most women's worries about food, rather than relating to changes and developments in nutritional thinking or specific diseases being linked to diet, centred on the highly publicised food scares of the time, such as those connected with red kidney beans and tinned salmon. This type of scare was mentioned by almost a third of women across the social spectrum. However, if it had led to a change in diet it was often only of a temporary nature; when the scare passed the food concerned returned to the table.

Most information on nutrition came from the mass media, and the differential use of the media might help to explain the different focus of concern expressed by women in different occupational classes. We found that 45% of women in classes I and II had listened to programmes related to food on BBC Radio 4, compared with 8% of women in class IIIN and no women from the other classes. A similar pattern was found for readership of 'quality' daily newspapers. Of women in classes I/II 45% read them compared with 9% in class IIIN, 7% in class IIIM and none in classes IV and V. Thus, middle-class women seemed to make much more use of the medium which was most likely to provide the most detailed coverage of nutritional issues; we are thinking of programmes such as 'The Food Programme' on Radio 4 and *The Guardian*'s coverage of this type of issue, particularly on what was then 'The Women's Page'.

Concern over the healthiness of food

Women also expressed concern about the types of things that were added to food, particularly processed and convenience foods, but fresh foods were also a cause for concern because of the liberal use of pesticides and herbicides.

I've not got a bee in my bonnet about it, but I do think a lot of what they put in food, that's not just tinned food, the stuff that they put on fresh foods now – the sprays and that – that worries me. I think we are getting a bit too free with the amount of stuff that's allowed to go on food. It does bother me to a certain extent but I wouldn't get fanatical about it.

This general uneasiness about food additives and sprays was widespread and only 33 (16%) of the women said that they had no worries at all about the food they ate. However, it was a general anxiety rather than a concern with *specific* dangers.

Even so, 70 (35%) of the women mentioned specific additives as giving cause for concern, mainly preservatives, colourings and flavourings; few mentioned sugar and hardly any were concerned about salt. In this context the lack of comprehensible labelling on foods was pointed to as something which prevented women from acting on their worries. The only way out of this impasse was thought to be the use of fresh foods, but even then there was the danger from the unfettered use of chemicals in modern agricultural production (Charles and Kerr, 1986b). Most women felt that as individuals they had no possibility of changing this situation so rather than worrying about it fruitlessly they shrugged it off:

I wouldn't say I worry about them [additives]. The fact that they have to give a list of what's in doesn't mean a thing to me because even if it's written on the packet or whatever – I mean I don't really know what it is. I'm not all that happy about it but, you know, I suppose you just have to trust that there's nothing awful going on . . . You sort of take it or leave it, don't you? I would say you either cooked all your own food and prepare all your own . . . but there again the vegetables that you buy have probably been sprayed with something or other.

And as one woman put it: 'There's a lot of things that I do think are worth changing but there's nowt I can do about it all no matter how hard you fight, so there's no use me getting uptight about it 'cos I'd make my life a misery and I'd make their life a misery.'

Most women felt impotent and powerless in the face of 'them' and 'their' control over what goes into food and how it is produced. To put it in other terms, when faced with the power of the food manufacturing industry and agribusiness to control the food available in the shops, exhortations to individual women to make their families' diets more healthy without, at the same time, exhorting the food producers not to produce food which is dangerous to health, seem designed to divert attention from those who have the power to change things and increase women's burden of anxiety and guilt. Their reaction, in most cases, is to ignore what they feel they cannot change unless it produces immediate and tangible effects.

If our hair was dropping out or we were getting very overweight while we were still eating what I would call sensibly, then I'd investigate the standards. There are of course people taking care of these things . . .

But I'm just generally aware of chemicals being mixed in with food rather than worrying.

Another important factor militating against health-conscious-ness is that it is commonly assumed that the family in general and, as we have seen, men in particular, will not be prepared to accept those foods which are perceived as being most healthy. As one woman said:

I would prefer to eat food that hasn't got a lot of things added but to do that you have to go to a health food shop and my husband wouldn't eat that type of food and I'm sure the kiddies wouldn't so I just plod along eating the things we've always eaten and just hope for the best.

These two factors meant that most women, even when they would have liked to change the family's diet so that it became more healthy, did not have the power to do so. They had to use foods which were available in the shops, which was determined by forces over which they felt they had no control, and to present the family with foods which were acceptable firstly to men and secondly to children. For the majority of women, providing food the family likes is the main consideration when deciding what to buy and make for a meal. Nutritional value comes a definite second, jostled by other factors such as cost and convenience. In fact 108 women (54%) said that the family's food preferences were their first consideration when deciding what to make for a meal. By contrast only 52 (26%) stated that they would place the nutritional value of food first and cost was almost as important being mentioned as the first consideration by 36 (18%) women. In the privil-eging of family preferences lies the realistic recognition that food that is disliked will not be eaten and food that is not eaten does no good at all: 'It's got to be something they like or they'll turn it away and they won't be getting any of the other things. They won't be getting filled up or goodness or anything.' Healthy eating, as well as being interpreted as eating a proper meal regularly, is also often viewed as something virtuous but not enjoyable. One woman speaks for many when she says: 'If you only did and ate and drank what people said is good for you, you'd lead a pretty miserable existence.' The notion that eating food that is good for you is hardly likely to be enjoyable may perhaps be traced back to many women's childhood experiences and their own mothers' attempts to get them to eat properly. Children are often encouraged to eat up food by being told it is good for them, as these women recall:

Liver was good for you. We got a lot of porridge when we were kids. The things you didn't like were good for you.

It always seemed the things you hated were good for you and the things you liked were bad for you.

The most common reason for eating food which women consider is not good in health terms is because it is liked by all. Sweets, cakes and biscuits were the most frequently mentioned foods in this category but foods high in fat content, such as chips and other fried food, were also frequently mentioned.

Families continue to eat these foods despite their unhealthy connotations because of the pleasure they afford, as this woman vividly describes:

I mean we like roast potatoes in the fat from the meat and in fact the marrow we had on Sunday was roasted round the meat and I love it like that. The flavour really comes from the juices in the meat but it's fatty and I'm very much aware of that but it's just lovely, it tastes so nice so we eat it. You've got to eat something you really enjoy haven't you? Whether or not it's beneficial or coated in cholesterol or whatever – there's got to be some pleasure, hasn't there. I think it should be a pleasurable time anyway, eating.

This woman was unusual in one respect. She regarded the Sunday roast as not being healthy. However, what characterises most of the foods described as being 'bad for you' is that they do not constitute part of a proper meal. A few women mentioned bread, meat and potatoes but they were much more commonly viewed as healthy foods, particularly meat, and the inclusion of bread and potatoes in the list can be understood as an indication of their 'fattening' properties. Foods which were 'fattening' were generally thought of as unhealthy but were, nevertheless, often eaten for the pleasure they afforded. This is explored in more detail in the next chapter, here we can note that the foods most women regarded as 'bad for you' were those commonly regarded as fattening.

'Eating properly'

When women talk about the contribution that food may make to health they characteristically talk about the importance of eating properly. The use of the term 'proper' is both significant and relevant to our discussion here for it is clear that proper eating, in terms of the consumption of proper meals at regular intervals, is taken by the majority of women to be equivalent to healthy eating. We asked all the women what they would prepare if they wanted to make a particularly healthy meal and most of them said they would cook a meal of meat, vegetables and potatoes; a proper meal. Of the women 80 (40%) stated unequivocally that a healthy meal would consist of meat and fresh vegetables and it featured in most other womens' series of alternatives. There was also evidence that a Sunday dinner was not only considered to be the proper meal par excellence, it was also the healthiest of meals: 'Well, I always think of meat and vegetables as being good for you so I suppose I would just do a traditional, maybe roast beef and plenty of vegetables and potatoes I think are fairly good for you.'

Proper meals and healthy meals are not only usually composed of meat or fish and vegetables, they are made from fresh ingredients. The vast majority of the women thought that fresh food was better for you than either frozen, tinned or packeted food. Only 16 women (8%) said there was no difference between fresh food and other foods and 132 (66%) felt that fresh food is better for you than either tinned or packeted food. A variety of reasons were put forward for espousing the greater benefits of fresh food when compared with other sorts of food. As well as the additives in tinned and packeted foods being of particular concern, the length of storage time was a worrying feature of frozen, tinned and packeted foods:

I suppose if you've no alternative it's [convenience food] better than nothing. It's probably just a question of taste on my part. But there's so much preservatives and such added to tinned food that I don't see how it can be as healthy. And the fact that they are stored for such a long time – same as frozen food – they must lose something.

There was also a strong feeling that all processing takes the goodness out of food. Fresh food has natural goodness; it's nearer to the natural source or so many women told us.

Processing, even in the form of freezing, can pervert this natural goodness and additives were a particular concern because they were not seen as natural. As one woman said: 'I mean it's not natural, so it can't be doing you any good.'

However, what seems to be crucial in determining the superior benefits of fresh food is the fact that it is cooked from scratch within the home. It is interesting that for some women, even the potentially perverting qualities of freezing do not apply when food is frozen at home by the woman herself: 22 women (11%) volunteered the view that if food was frozen at home this was as good as fresh but the same could not be said of commercially frozen food. This may be partly because women see themselves as having more control over such food; they prepare it therefore they know what's in it and how long they've had it. But home cooking from fresh ingredients has a moral as well as nutritional value, it is part of being a good wife and mother. One woman, for example said:

Well, you probably don't need meat every day but I have this sort of fixed thing you must have meat, vegetables ... I suppose when I do meals like fish fingers, baked beans and chips I feel guilty, I don't know why, I always think they're not having a good dinner here.

The feeling that home preparation guarantees or, at least, lends goodness to food is also displayed in women's definition of what constitutes junk food. Packeted or instant foods which only require the addition of water before serving, ready-prepared foods such as beefburgers and fish fingers, and takeaways are all commonly nominated as junk food. There is a straightforward concern with nutritional value in the definition of food as junk, for example, sweets, crisps and carbonated drinks are also likely to be seen as junk food and some women define such food simply as that which has no nutritional value. Nevertheless, the mode of preparation definitely emerges as a significant consideration in women's evaluations and many women describe convenience food as filling you up without doing you any good. One woman simply said: 'At the moment I think of junk food as anything which is ready made.'

For another woman it appeared clear that good food has to be worked at and while convenience foods are a useful standby if one is short of time, such consumption does not constitute eating properly or healthily.

All this packet junk is . . . I mean, it's just not true. How can something cook in two minutes that's supposed to be something that's fresh and healthy for you? No, I don't think it's healthy but you do have them in . . . I mean if you haven't much time and it's 'Oh well, they can have that tonight, I haven't much time' but if I'd all the time in the world just to devote to cooking it would be all proper stuff.

These sort of feelings were echoed in many other women's descriptions of junk food and it becomes clear that certain food items, such as beefburgers, can be nutritious if cooked at home but may be regarded as junk food if bought ready-prepared as convenience food or ready-cooked as a takeaway.

Things you can buy from a shop and either chuck in the oven or in a tin heat up neat, so virtually everything in the freezers in the shops apart from vegetables, y'know frozen chips, frozen chicken, pies, etc. And tinned ready dinners. And snackpots, etc. Absolutely revolting I should think. I mean hamburgers I suppose are the obvious ones but I think if they're cooked nicely and home-made they're absolutely delicious. But tinned hamburgers, frozen hamburgers are y'know.

Beefburgers, pizzas – they wouldn't be junk if I made them myself, but I'm not keen on any frozen food.'

Convenience foods

It is interesting at this point to look a little more closely at the nature of convenience foods and the way that women assess their 'goodness'. Convenience foods come in many forms from instant coffee and tea bags to Snack Pots and Pot Noodles. Even meat that is not 'proper' meat, such as sausages, is regarded as a convenience food. In fact, it seems that any food which has had work performed on it outside the home, such that it is no longer fresh, and that will save time in its preparation and cooking inside the home can be regarded as convenience food. Thus the way food is categorised depends not so much on the end product, perhaps a beefburger, but on the process of production that a certain food has undergone and who has performed work on it. This is crucial. If a woman (hardly ever a man) has performed work inside the home on mince and the other ingredients which she bought fresh, and has produced a beefburger then it is not classified as convenience food. If, on the other hand, this work has been carried out by a butcher or a food manufacturing company then the beefburger – even if it contained identical ingredients – would be regarded as convenience food. The labour time expended on the production of convenience food is usually expended outside the home under a different system of social relations. The labour time of the 'housewife' is thereby reduced. It would seem therefore that any food which saves time in meal preparation within the home is regarded as a convenience food. This is the case even when it is not specifically marketed as such. Frozen and tinned foods such as frozen peas and tinned fruit are no exception to this rule. Frozen peas require no shelling and tinned oranges require no peeling. Frozen meat may perhaps seem to be anomalous but it can be argued that buying meat and storing it in a freezer reduces the amount of time women need to spend in shopping. Fresh meat would probably necessitate a daily shopping trip whereas frozen meat reduces the need for frequent visits to the butcher.

Convenience foods also enable people to eat fruit and vegetables that are not in season, strawberries are available all the year round, thus divorcing food production from 'nature' and the natural cycles of the year. Convenience food is also in some way food that is not natural or fresh, two concepts very closely linked in the women's attitudes towards food. Because of this rupture with what is natural and good (healthy) and because there is less time required for the preparation of convenience food, it is generally not considered to be as good for you as fresh food. Expending time and effort on the production of a meal in some way conferred goodness on it; perhaps a moral rather than nutritional goodness but this distinction was not made by the women. In addition, food that required time to be expended on its preparation and cooking usually ended up as part of a proper meal, which was by definition good for you. Meals made up of convenience foods, such as sausages and baked beans, were not in the same class as proper meals. And many women expressed guilt that they had to resort to convenience foods, particularly, possibly only, if a *main* meal consisted of convenience foods. Ideally, therefore, women felt that preparing meals using fresh ingredients was best but in practice, for a multitude of reasons, things did not always work out that way. Practically *all* the women we spoke to used convenience foods in one form or another during the diary fortnight. One woman sometimes used tins of meatballs:

If I've been in a rush or had a bad day or been out I do that for a convenient meal. If I've had a bad day with the baby and he's really been fretting, teething, and I've nursed him all day, I find it's just as easy to open that tin. I mean I know it's not right but some days you have to ... When you've had a baby you tend to do more convenience ... 'cos you don't have the time that you'd like to have ... to sit down and think what should I do?

She clearly felt guilty that circumstance led her to resort to convenience foods.

Guilt was often associated with the use of convenience foods, usually because not enough time had been spent preparing a 'proper' meal for the family:

I suppose when I do meals like fish fingers and baked beans and chips I feel guilty – I don't know why – I always think that they're not having a very good dinner here. I suppose I do think about it subconsciously and try to give them something that's healthy for tea.

The guilt, we would suggest, arises because of the close association in women's minds between a proper meal and a healthy meal. A meal consisting of convenience foods which, as we have seen, cannot constitute a proper meal, is by definition less healthy than a proper meal and involves much less preparation time. Women therefore feel guilty when, through force of circumstance, they take the easy way out and do not spend time and effort preparing and cooking a proper healthy meal: 'Sometimes if there's been a lot going on and we've had convenience foods, sort of tins and things, I think "Oh dear, we should have had more fresh meat and veg this week", you know, "all these additives and things", but that's as far as it goes.' Interestingly, when women spoke about their use of convenience food they almost always referred to their inclusion, or otherwise, in the main meal of the day. The non-main meal in many households frequently consisted of convenience foods but this was not seen as problematic in the way that their inclusion in the main meal was. 'Well I do go for a few convenience foods now I've got the children, it's easier if I'm going out anywhere for just a quick snack at lunch time.'

This resort to convenience foods was regarded as an innovation that was unheard of in their mother's day. Indeed, ideas of nutritional goodness associated with home cooking and proper eating seem, at least partly, to owe their existence to women's memories of their own childhoods. One woman expresses this very clearly when she says: 'I suppose convenience food I call junk food mostly because I suppose I have this inbuilt thing from home that anything you prepare from scratch is better for you.'

A great many women said that they cooked similar meals to those their mothers prepared for them as children and it seems that mothers are an important source of information when women begin to feed their own families. In fact, 90 women (45%) said that they cook the same sort of meals as their mothers used to and 83 women (42%) mentioned their mothers as the most helpful source of information on feeding a family. At the same time it was not uncommon for women to remark that their own meal provision was inferior to that of their mothers because the latter always cooked from scratch whereas they themselves use more convenience foods. Most mothers are reported to have cooked proper meals from fresh ingredients and, as such, were 'lovely cooks'.

My mum was a lovely cook, she used to always bake – bake every week, it was lovely. Always lovely meals. On a lunch-time when I used to come home from school there was always a proper meal on the table and a pudding as well . . . she used to make everything, baking was always fresh and it was lovely.

My mother was a lovely cook, she used to cook more than I do. She'd cook meat and two veg and a pudding. We don't have puddings. She used to cook like that, pudding and two veg and always meat every day.

The centrality of the proper meal to this conception of home cooking is brought out in these comments. Home baking and soup making were also skills that mothers commonly possessed and practised and women often lamented that they themselves did not possess such talents. This homely cooking is sometimes seen as having generally passed into history or is associated with rural life; accounts of the goodness of such food are redolent with sentimentality but are nevertheless strongly felt. The conviction that home made soup, for example, has great goodness is shown in the fact that many women make soup when family members are ill although soup may otherwise be bought in tins and packets. Of the women 98 (49%) said that soup was eaten in illness. One women said:

I tend to give people more soups and more hot drinks rather than solid things and I do make the effort then to make my own soup rather than taking a packet out of the cupboard. I think there's a lot more food in home made soup, you get proper veggies and things.

We may therefore see women's concern that the family should eat properly and healthily in terms of home cooked food provided at regular intervals as having been handed down through family tradition; it is a central part of family life.

A common feature of mothers' cooking which does not, however, seem to have been inherited by the majority of women is a concern with filling the family up. Some women describe their mother's cooking thus: 'Anything in vast quantities was always good for you and it would always build you up. Steamed pudding and custard was a preference, I think. My mum was all for getting you fed up, and if you were fed up, you were fine.' Ensuring the family is 'fed up' now appears an outdated concept based on the experience of want although it may still constitute a decision-making factor for women managing on low incomes. Concern is now more likely to be expressed about family members who eat too much and many foods are regarded as not being good for you to eat simply because they are fattening.

The weight factor

In fact a further significant feature of the way in which women talk about diet and its relation to health is the striking congruence between ideas about healthy eating and ideas about slimming. Thus, the foods most frequently mentioned as being healthy – fresh meat with fresh vegetables, fresh fruit and salads – are those which women most commonly say they eat when they are on a diet, and the foods most often cited as being bad for you – sweet foods, fried foods, bread and potatoes in large quantity – are those which women avoid when they are on a diet. This is not mere coincidence for it is apparent that for many women a good diet is taken to be equivalent to dieting. In fact, some women assumed that when we began to talk to them about diet what we meant was dieting, as the following exchange between inter- viewer and respondent indicates:

[Do you think there are certain foods that are essential to *your* daily diet? I mean we talked before about what you thought was important for Adam [son] to eat, do you think there are certain things which are important for yourself to eat?] I just eat anything me. Food's important to me. I couldn't diet. No way could I diet. Mark's mum [mother-in-law] diets a lot.

There are good reasons for this confusion in terminology when we reflect on the sources from which many women gain information on diet.

Firstly, we might consider their experience with health care advisers. Overweight is the major reason for talking to general practitioners about diet and for consulting dieticians, but it is also true to say that women's contact with preventive health care services is likely to encourage them to lay emphasis on weight as the primary concern in the regulation of diet. The ante-natal clinic and the child health clinic emerge as the places where mothers are most likely to encounter professional advice on diet although such advice is commonly viewed as inadequate and not related to the concerns women experience in feeding a family. What is evident about both these sources of information is that a great deal of emphasis is placed on weight as an evaluation of both a healthy pregnancy and a healthy child. Diet does not seem likely to be discussed unless weight is an issue and remonstrations to reduce weight are rarely accompanied by much explanation. This is worth exploring in some detail.

Advice on diet is an accepted part of care for a healthy pregnancy but most women could not recall being given verbal advice on their own eating habits, although some information was available in the leaflets that women receive in the ante-natal clinic. Some women clearly regretted that there had been no opportunity to discuss dietary issues and would have appreciated clearer guidelines for practice. Others recalled being told to eat 'a balanced diet' or the 'right things' but did not receive any information on what these might be. The assumption that women know what these terms mean is clearly not justified. One woman's comments were typical:

They told me to keep my weight down, that was all. They didn't give me a diet or anything. It was difficult. Didn't mean anything really. I would rather they'd given me a sheet saying, look, these are the best things for you to eat. There was no time to discuss things which might have been more helpful.

Some women however felt the advice had been helpful. One said:

Only through having children they've told you what was good for you
and they give you all these leaflets and things – especially for
breastfeeding to make your milk better I suppose . . . And so of course
I'd taken that to heart when I was feeding Julie, like liver and milk and
fish and cheese.

Some women commented that the advice they had been given
was merely common sense. But the nature of this common sense
seems to vary widely with different aspects of diet being recalled
by different women. Some women recalled the importance of
milk intake which had been impressed upon them; others
emphasised fruit and vegetable consumption. Protein and iron
received attention from others and some concentrated on low
carbohydrate intake. While all these aspects do bear some
relation to advice they might have been given during pregnancy
the lack of any summation of all these factors in the women's
accounts, plus the evidence that no two women came up with the
same combination of dietary features, suggests a very jumbled
picture of nutritional information. Some typical comments are
included below for the purposes of illustration:

They just said to eat plenty of protein and not to eat too many
carbohydrates, not to eat white bread and things like that.
Just eat the right foods; fresh fruit and vegetables, a balanced diet.
They told me to eat plenty of red meat and to take my iron tablets.
I was told to eat liver and pulses and to generally eat well.

From almost all their accounts it seems that the advice
particularly emphasises weight watching. Women continually
made reference to the fact that they were told to keep an eye on
their weight and yet they also felt they were not given the
necessary nutritional information to do this.

They moan if you put weight on. They moan if you don't put enough on.
They never bothered to give you a diet or anything. And I thought
afterwards, really, it's not right, there should be a diet there for them to
give you, to help you because lots of people do put an awful lot of weight
on and it's not 'cos of eating too much, it's just not eating the right
things for the body to cope with.

Even women who had made a positive evaluation of the advice
they had received drew our attention to the importance placed

on weight by professional advisers: 'They say that if you keep to a reasonable diet you won't put on so much weight and if you control your weight it'll be easier to lose it later on. I found that reassuring.' This concentration on weight seems to be a feature of clinic procedures and takes material form in the practice of regularly weighing pregnant women to assess progress and to check on their health. While this may be an important exercise in itself, it seems to lead to a situation where weight becomes the only reason for discussing diet. This may engender feelings of guilt and reinforces women's continually existing concern with their weight; in addition it appears to deny the possibility of a more holistic approach to diet and eating habits. These practices serve to confirm many women's beliefs that adequate nutrition is equivalent to slimness and that a good diet means dieting and controlling weight.

It was not only the women's weight which was monitored: the weight of their babies, once they were born, seemed to be the focus of the health care professionals' concern. The women often recalled distressing incidents which centred on their child's weight. One woman told us:

And they fussed over Ruth's weight, I mean they even brought me from the clinic a pair of scales. She was gaining weight but just 'cos I happened to mention I was worried in me mind, was she getting enough feed 'cos she wasn't contented, you know I was test-weighing her before each feed in these little scales, writing it down – it was all so traumatic at the time.

And another said:

At the clinic she started to lose weight. First she wasn't putting much on and then she started to lose it and the health visitor at the clinic and my health visitor kept saying 'Oh, it's because you haven't got enough milk.' They said I'd got to put her on the bottle . . . I tried her with it but she didn't like the bottle either and for about two weeks she was hardly getting anything . . . I couldn't get it through to the health visitor about how difficult it was . . . when I first started telling them at the clinic I burst into tears and I think they thought I was neurotic or something.

It seems crystal clear from the women's accounts that, as with advice during pregnancy, weight is the central issue in relation to much infant feeding advice. At the child health clinic women were not usually offered advice on feeding if their children's weight was seen to be appropriate for their age. Thus good feeding was understood solely in terms of weight gains and losses.

Well I did take him down to the clinic. It's only once a fortnight and I don't think they said anything about food, unless perhaps he'd been putting weight on. They assumed that because he was putting weight on he'd be getting the right sort of thing.

And if a child's weight was increasing normally this could invalidate other concerns:

I felt fed up with the health visitors 'cos they did seem to straightaway get her on to the bottle and not try to sort out the problem. With Stephen as well he never used to put sort of the exact amount on each week. All they seemed to be bothered about was whether he was putting weight on all the time.

Great emphasis was placed on the weight of children in their early months and weight loss or weight gain could result in women's feeding practice and their maternal competence being called into question:

They started telling me not to feed so much . . . 'cos he was a fat baby. He's not now. He's tall and slim. They kept telling me off that he was getting fat so I stopped going.

I was actually asked 'Are you feeding him enough or are you holding him back because you want him to be slim like you?' . . . After he was one I haven't taken him because I thought there's no point if they're going to carry on saying he's underweight. I can't force him to eat food, if he won't eat it, he won't eat it . . . I thought 'Gosh, he's not the weight he should be, I'd better get something down him.' But again, my health visitor said I'd done very well and although he hasn't gained the amount he should have done in the six months or twelve months there's nothing wrong with him, he's strong and healthy and kicking, so don't worry. But at the clinic they seemed to be saying I should worry.

Such criticism of their babies was viewed very negatively by the women and often stopped them attending clinics. It could even affect women's practice at second hand: 'My sister-in-law went and she got told off about the baby's weight and I thought that nobody is going to tell me off so I didn't bother going.' These and similar comments reveal the lack of utility of this form of approach as well as the distress that it undoubtedly causes to the women who experience such criticism.

As we have seen, women based *their* evaluation of adequate nutrition on whether their children appeared healthy or not and they pointed out that the 'fat babies make fat children' view which some professional advisers seemed to promote bore no relation to their own experience:

She advised me to keep off puddings because he was so big. But I thought it was silly really because he was going to lose weight once he starts moving around. I still give him puddings every now and again. I went completely against her advice and he doesn't look so bad on it.

Once again, we would make the point that a concentration on weight as an indicator of feeding practice not only denies the importance of other indicators, such as the observation of a child as alert and active, but obscures the more general connections to be made between diet and health and denies the possibility of a holistic approach to eating habits. In this context it is hardly surprising that women's views of the goodness or otherwise of foods seems to bear a remarkable similarity to those foods they regard as 'fattening'. Health care professionals seem to reinforce women's obsession with food and weight and in addition to the concentration of health care professionals on weight many women seem to base their ideas of nutrition on slimming literature. This undoubtedly affects their attitudes to diet and health more generally. Sometimes it means that a varied diet will be espoused because women have had such bad experiences with weight-reducing diets which place an emphasis on consumption of one particular food, but more often it results in the under-valuation of foods such as bread and potatoes which are seen as fattening. More significantly, perhaps, it can engender feelings that consciousness about diet takes all the pleasure out of eating, for most women find slimming a miserable experience, thus adding to the feeling that healthy eating is virtuous but unenjoyable.

In this chapter we have shown that women's conceptions of healthy eating owe more to social categories and values than to nutritional and other supposedly scientific values. Within a system of classification and understanding based on social processes they feel responsible for ensuring that their families eat properly, although their own food needs are not always given enough attention to prevent women themselves becoming worn out and run down. Food is felt to be important to health, certain foods are 'better for you' than others, and these are usually foods which constitute part of a proper, family diet. Other foods, for a variety of reasons, are not considered to be either proper or healthy. Thus, although women may show a certain wariness of nutritional experts, and may not alter their families' diets according to the latest nutritional trends, they take their responsibility for their families' health very seriously indeed, and do their utmost to ensure that they are eating properly.

7

Women and food: friend or enemy?

In this chapter we focus on women's own relationship to food: a relationship which is essentially contradictory and problematic. When women are looking after young children and are at home for much of the day, food, its provision and preparation, is a major preoccupation. Women are concerned to feed their children properly and this means preparing three meals a day, thinking about what they will eat and enjoy, and making sure that they eat it. Food needs to be prepared for men; it needs to be presented in the form of a proper meal which is acceptable to adults and children alike, and men may have packed lunches made for them and are usually provided with breakfast before they leave for work in the morning. Even at the level of venturing outside the confines of the home, it is shopping for food which often provides the only pretext for an outing in the day. As one woman succinctly described it: 'If you're a mother, food obviously takes a very big part of your day up because if you're not shopping you're preparing it and then you're eating it and cleaning up after it.' In between meals there are likely to be 'snacks', food such as biscuits and sweets and, less frequently, fruit, often eaten not just to satisfy appetite but as a means of providing a break in the day for both women and children. Food is constantly within reach at home in ways that it is not in a more structured work situation, so as well as being on women's minds it is easily available for the occasional (or frequent) nibble. In addition to these material circumstances which place women in almost constant contact with food, women are concerned to achieve or maintain a slim, attractive body image. They are with food all day, feeding others, but most of those we spoke to felt at the same time that they must deny food to themselves.

The complexity of women's relationship to food was brought out in a series of questions we asked them about their feelings about their own weight. In many cases there was enormous guilt and anxiety attached to food and eating which often related to their situation at home, financially dependent on their partners, and with young, demanding children requiring constant care and attention. Food was viewed as a treacherous friend by many women: they desired it for the pleasure it gave but denied themselves the pleasure because of the unacceptable weight gain that might result if they indulged themselves. At the same time it was a comfort, a support in time of need, but again a comfort which had a sting in the tail – penalties of weight gain were paid for turning to food. Women therefore find themselves in a contradictory situation as regards food and their feelings about it are ambivalent and problematic. One woman, who had recently had a baby, described the situation as follows:

It's a vicious circle. If I feel I'm overweight I get upset so I eat 'cos I *hate* being overweight, it really upsets me, I hate it. It's all tied in with having a baby as well because – because I've had a baby I don't want to look frumpy or old so obviously it's important to have a nice figure so that you are not going to look old and horrible and everything, but because I'm slightly overweight I eat then to comfort myself. I mean even though I'm sat here telling you this and I know I do it but after all I can't stop myself doing it, I still do it and then I feel terrible afterwards. After I've done it, you know, I'll have a mad binge, and then I feel so utterly desolate after I've finished, I think 'You stupid fool.' Then I go and do the same thing the next day because I think, 'Well I've already done it the day before so I'm off my diet anyway.' It's stupid . . . [laughs] I know it's there but I can't stop it, I can't break into it. But if I start to lose some, say by accident like now and I've not actually been dieting, it encourages me and usually I can go on and on and on but if I have . . . if I go out on a night out and I eat a meal then I start again because I think I've broken my diet you see. Perhaps I'm mad.

This 'madness' is something that she shares, to a greater or lesser extent, with the majority of the women we spoke to and it indicates the precarious balancing act continually being performed by women to retain control over their food intake and, through that, over their bodies. It also points to the fact that eating disorders, such as anorexia nervosa or compulsive eating, are not so far removed from women's so-called normal relationship to food. In fact, several of the women suffered from one or other of these eating disorders, and the feelings they expressed – about themselves and about food – were echoed in the accounts of all the women.

The dissatisfaction of women with their bodies, which seems to us to underly this contradictory and problematic relationship to food, was widespread in our sample. For example only 23 of the women (11·5%) had never dieted or been worried about their weight, although 48 (24%) of them said that they were now happy with or resigned to their present weight; 68 (34%) of the women said they were either dieting or watching their weight at the time of interview, and for many of them this weight consciousness had become so much a part of their eating patterns that it hardly merited a mention. One woman told us that she became obsessed with eating if she followed a diet, she therefore did not diet. 'I think it's far better to have sensible eating habits from being young . . . and then you don't ever really have that problem.' However, it was clear that her food intake had been adapted to maintain an acceptable weight, so in this sense she was dieting:

I did alter my eating habits so I try and keep to – I don't eat as many chips or potatoes as I would have done years ago, but it's just normal for me 'cos I'm used to having small portions of chips. At one time I did actually have about three on my plate and then craved for them all night whereas now I have a smaller helping and I feel as though I've not been cheated.

For many women the questions on dieting seemed to release a flood of dissatisfaction and guilt, not only with their bodies and their weight but with their whole social situation. This related to many areas of their lives: having a baby, getting married, giving up work, sexual attractiveness, retaining the affection and sexual interest of a partner. These are all fundamental issues and problems which arise from the structural position of women in our society (ideologically defined as dependants of men) and the contradictory ideologies of motherhood and fulfilment through maternity, on the one hand, and female sexual attractiveness involving the maintenance of unrealistically slim bodies and continual self-denial as far as food is concerned, on the other. This response to questions of diet seems to indicate that food is fundamentally tied in with women's feelings about themselves and about the social world they inhabit. Three such responses illustrate this point. One woman had just had a baby, her first, and now had a weight problem. She turns to food at times of stress:

What I do is if I've had a bad day or if I'm nervous – I eat when I'm nervous and it's always been a failing of mine. And since I've had Sally I can't control it. I'm hoping that when she gets older it'll be easier to manage but I started smoking to help, to try to smoke instead of eat, but it does work to a certain point but – I know it's not good for me so I try not to smoke too many. So I don't always fall back on cigarettes – I'll fall back on food and as a result I'm about a stone overweight than what I was before I had Sally 'cos she is a source of tension – a great source of tension. [So you eat . . . it's just having Sally really that's . . .] Oh, definitely. I didn't cope well with her at all really. It started there on and it's not been easy to give up and she's still . . . I'm just not the type to take to motherhood easily. I wanted her, we planned for her, but when she arrived she was a shock to me – I didn't know what she'd be like. I mean I didn't expect it and she really gets on my nerves so I eat.

Another woman found that moving and getting married had affected her relationship to food and she explained this as a result of depression. She was asked if she was happy with her present weight and told us:

I don't mind at the present time, I have been a couple of stone heavier than I am at present and that was when I first got married when we used to eat a lot more chips and things really. I think it was a depressive thing with me in actual fact that put my weight on when I first got married really because I lived away from home and I think I ate through depression. I think I was not just homesick but 'friendsick' as well really – sort of people that we'd known we missed. Moving into a completely different environment and getting married and everything else, different place to work, everything changed at once and it just depressed me for the first few weeks – first year in particular and that's when I put all the weight on in the first year I got married really and then over the next year or two I gradually managed to get it back down again.

For another woman eating was intimately bound up with her not having a job and the unsatisfactory relationship she had with her partner. Her relationship to food was linked to feelings of self-confidence and control over her own social situation. She described what had happened when she'd got married, given up work and had a child:

We started off wrongly and it was his money, his house, and it tended to be his food as well so I just didn't eat, I'd eat what I could off the family allowance ... I was totally ... nothing. No self-confidence, nothing was mine, I was there for the use of. [And how have you got round that?] Went back to work – my independence, that's why I always work.

Why women diet

These women's experiences illustrate how complex women's relationship to food is and how much it is implicated in their overall social situation and the social relationships in which they find themselves. We can begin unravelling the nature of this relationship by exploring the reasons given by women for needing or wanting to diet, most of which seem to be linked to notions of sexuality and attractiveness. However, as we can see from the experiences of the three women just quoted, food is tied up with feelings of self worth in other ways also; and wishing to remain sexually alluring, particularly to the partners on whom women are financially dependent at this stage in the life cycle, can also be understood in this way. This is particularly true when we consider that feelings of self-confidence can often be reinforced or, conversely, undermined by the approval or disapproval of men. Many women told us of their partner's comments about their weight or shape when they were asked about their dissatisfaction with their bodies; and it should be noted that dissatisfaction did not only occur if women felt themselves to be overweight. It could also arise from being too 'skinny' or not having enough 'up top'.

One woman told us:

Well, sometimes I feel as though I could be a bit bigger, a bit fatter. Only because Dave goes on about it all the time ... he doesn't like bony women. He'd prefer me to be a bit fatter. He likes me when I've just – for example when I've just had a baby 'cos I'm pretty big, you know. He likes you to be well covered ...

And another told us of her feelings about her 'fatness':

I mean I'm conscious of it [weight] when I put clothes on that feel uncomfortable that used to feel all right, I'm talking about dresses and things that I've had for a number of years, you know ... and my husband notices and says 'You're getting a bit round there'. I tend to put a lot on round my bottom and my legs, you know, 'I'd cut out that chocolate if I were you.'

And another spoke of the ability of men to undermine women's confidence in themselves:

I'd like to lose about half a stone but knowing me I'd probably lose it in all the wrong places anyway, so I'll just stick to what I've got. In the summer when you're wearing thinner things all your bulges show don't they, so you're more conscious of it really. I'm all right until he says 'Look at your fat bottom', or something like that and then you think 'Oh God!', you know, 'perhaps I should try to lose weight or something'. They really do wonders to boost your morale. You can't really say much to them can you? I mean, he's getting hold of you and saying 'Look at all this fat here', and there's nothing on him that you can get anywhere near.

Even men's comments about fatness in general affected women's views of their own bodies:

Oh, I'd hate to be fat – I just would hate it. I mean if I get over eight stone now I cut down for a couple of days just to get back down to eight or just under. I mean I know when Graham sees fat people he'll say 'How on earth do they let themselves get into that state in the first place?' I don't think he'd want to stay with me if I was fat. And I don't like to see fat people myself.

This last comment indicates the cultural attitudes towards 'fatness' in our society. It is something which is disapproved of and is almost judged in moral terms, someone who is fat has 'let themselves go' and they earn social disapproval. They are, significantly, no longer regarded as attractive, particularly in sexual terms. The concern to maintain sexual attractiveness through conforming to the ideal body image of slimness was brought out again and again by the women. It was not only regarded as an important way of ensuring that your partner stayed with you, but it also boosted women's confidence to be made aware – by men – that they were considered sexually attractive. The following account illustrates this point vividly:

I do feel a lot better, lighter. I mean I've been at nine and a half stone and I know what I felt like and also when I got to that weight I had jeans which I've never really let myself wear 'cos I know what I'd look like in jeans because I always tended to be heavy legged anyway – I got rid of most of that when I got to that weight and I felt very well. David thought I looked very well – you see that's a lot of it as well I think. [Does he encourage you to lose weight then?] Yes, he does. I also know that when we used to live in town and I used to take Alan out in a pushchair and I'd go past workmen in town and I used to get whistled at and that really boosted my ego somewhat because that's never really happened to me and I'd got to this magical weight and it was tremendous, you know, people were suddenly taking notice of this wonderful slim me. [So you're missing getting all those whistles?] I am,

I am missing that. I'm missing Dave's compliments. I don't get complimented like I used to and I'm missing those clothes. As well I know it's bad for me to be like I am. I can tell just . . . I mean doing housework and that, I mean I'm not so overweight that I can't do housework without getting out of breath, you know, I can run after Alan and things like that but I know myself from just going out for a run – I think 'God, at twenty eight I should be able to do a bit better than this', you know, and it is just with being too heavy.

Men, whether partners, men on the streets, or even boys at school, are vital in reinforcing women's feelings about the need to remain slim. On this latter point one woman said:

I think when you go to school, secondary school, when you start getting interested in clothes you start to think 'Why am I fatter than her?', and sort of get aware of yourself. Boys are cruel, 'Ugh, look at her isn't she fat!' . . . you know what they're like. Then you take a long look at yourself and you think you could do to lose it.

Clearly, an interest in slimming begins from a very early age. Many of the women spoke of their attempts to slim when they were at school and of the inevitability of girls becoming interested in dieting around puberty. This, of course, is the time when sexuality and sexual attractiveness begin to concern girls. One woman described her experience as a young teenager:

I think you go through stages . . . when you're sort of a teenager and girls go through this stage where you can't be plump and you find that you live on lettuce leaves – I tried that once – I fainted that many times at school . . . I just went through this stage where I just thought I was absolutely fat and I wanted to be a size ten and my Mum said that if you were a size ten anyway the dress would be half way up your legs 'cos you're not exactly the original size to be a size ten. My mother's a bit of a scream, she took it all in good part, she was worried but she sort of laughed it off until I got some sense, I've got some somewhere. [How long did you last just eating lettuces?] I don't know – about six months I would say by the time I'd finished, except you'd go through the stage when you'd last a few weeks and then you'd go on a binge, you know, I think we were all doing it at school at the time – how thin we were. I should think that the fashion at that stage was that you had to be that thin.

She was still concerned about her weight mainly because of her appearance and fitting into fashionable clothes. This concern with appearance and sexual attractiveness is promoted and exploited by commercial interests. Holidays in the sun and the images of bronzed bikini-clad bodies often prompted women to slim at the beginning of summer when all their unwanted 'bulges' were in danger of being exposed. One woman, who never ate bread or sweet things because of her propensity to gain weight, told us that she had been in town one day:

I was looking at some of the diet plans in Boots the other day, looking at this picture of a wonderful lissom lady lying on a beach and thinking 'Gosh, maybe I ought to look like that for the summer!' – then I started to look at the prices and they were terrific.

There is clearly a big profit to be made out of promoting abnormal female slenderness which commercial interests have been quick to take up. As one of the women wryly commented, you must need 'a heck of a lot of money to slim properly.'

Slimness is particularly associated with beaches in exotic faraway places, fast cars, alcohol, palm trees and young sexually alluring men and women. This lifestyle is fostered by commercial interests largely through the fashion industry and advertising and is something to which many women aspire. One of the women we interviewed had been anorexic, and it was lying on a beach in a sunny holiday resort abroad that had triggered off her experience:

Well, I got this job, I was seventeen in the December and in the March I got this job nannying in London. I'd always been plump and my sister was so skinny, she could eat anything. I did eat an awful lot, an awful lot of fish and chips and I was overweight, especially as I am so small. She used to call me 'Barrel Features' and I used to call her 'String Bean' and we were always arguing. Anyway, I got this job and went down to London and in the last week of May, first week of June, they were going . . . on holiday. Well of course it was paid for me to go as well, so off I went. Well, when I was out there there was all the girls, women, walking round in bikinis. Well, I felt . . . suddenly after all the carrying on my sister had at me saying 'Lose weight, lose weight!', it hadn't sunk in, I'd laughed at her, couldn't care less. Then it really sunk in to me and I kept thinking 'Oh my God!', and so I started it there.

This is interesting, because although the apparent trigger for her anorexia was seeing other women in bikinis and feeling that she had to emulate their slimness, it also coincided with her being away from home for the first time, an event which has been implicated in the onset of anorexia by some authors. The sexual dimension of the slimming business is highlighted by a recent experience that also arose from her continuing dissatisfaction with her body. Her anorexia had been so severe that eventually she had had to undergo psychiatric treatment in hospital during which she decided that she may as well eat again. She was asked if she was now happy with her weight:

I am, apart from the fact that I'm top heavy which is something that I found before – that it was only when I got under seven stone that I could lose it from there. Maybe it's since having children that it's a bit more difficult to lose it from there. I know that for a lot of people that's the first place they lose it from, and they are always moaning and saying 'Oh I lose it from there'. It's the last for me, I can lose it from down here which a lot of people find difficult but it's just my bust . . . it used to get me depressed a lot and I went to see a doctor who said that I could have had it on the National Health to make it smaller. He told me about what they'd do – scars here, etc. – so I went home and I sat down and thought about it and I thought, well it's not nature, it didn't seem right to me to go to that extreme – I kept thinking about all these things they do to people like making them bigger and making them smaller and I thought that surely later in life when your body changes I could imagine that something drastic was going to happen. I thought that you might be in pain so I just got to thinking that it wasn't worth it, it was just one of those things that I'd have to learn to live with. It was just like – people wear these halter necks or go bra-less when it's something that I can't do, and I often can see him ogling at – and it used to . . . now he knows that it was upsetting me and he's not that bothered and, you know, he was very good and he said it didn't bother him, but it did me, you know – well there's always something to moan about isn't there.

Many women were clearly unhappy about their own weight because they felt that a slimmer shape *must* be more attractive. The extent to which this feeling is fostered directly by the men in their lives may vary but most attend to the dominant cultural view of 'slim is beautiful' which is given significant emphasis in women's magazines and mass advertising.

Given the medical profession's concern with obesity, it was striking that a relatively low number of women gave consider-ations of health as a reason for their dissatisfaction with their weight. In fact, 43 (21·5%) of the women mentioned a concern for health as being among the reasons for dieting although only 8 (4%) mentioned health as the sole reason. In contrast, 80 (40%) mentioned their appearance and 55 (27·5%) mentioned fitting into their clothes. The tenuous nature of the concern for health can be gauged from the type of response to the question of why dieting was important. A typical comment was 'So my clothes will fit me. I do feel a lot better, as well.' This *could* be

interpreted as showing a concern for health, but it may be more
likely to reflect a sense of well-being arising from the confidence
of knowing yourself to be slim and therefore attractive and
desirable. Another typical comment was 'Just to get some
weight down – all that flab looks revolting. And I suppose you
feel better.' In addition only 6 (3%) of the women obtained their
diet from health care professionals. And indeed one of the
women who had been advised to lose weight by her doctor did
not feel that her main reason for wanting to lose weight was to
become more healthy:

Vanity, that's all it is. Really, I should diet 'cos I've got trouble with my
leg. I think it does help varicose veins if you're not carrying a lot of
weight and that's one reason why, really, I should. If you put too much
weight on it's bad for your heart, they say, you've got a better chance of
dying young if you're fat. I don't know how true it is because there's a
lot of fat people walking about aren't there? No, with me it's more
vanity really – being vain I suppose. I don't like to think of it like that,
but that's what it is.

The contradictions of self-denial

Most of the women therefore denied themselves certain sorts of
foods in the interests of maintaining their sexual attractiveness
and retaining their partners. At the same time, however, they
had to feed their partners and children 'properly' ensuring that
the children grew and developed healthily and that the men
were refuelled so that they returned to work well fed and
contented. The self-denial involved in dieting and weight
watching was therefore taking place in a social context in
which healthy, nutritious food had to be prepared and provided
for others. Differing ideologies of femininity here come into
conflict. As one women said 'It is difficult to be a mother and a
lover at the same time': the demands on women are contradictory and often irreconcilable. This contradiction was clearly
voiced by one of the women:

I started dieting when I was breast feeding – everyone said you
shouldn't do that, you must not try to lose weight when you're breast
feeding – 'cos I was so fat after I'd had him. I'd put on three stone and I
only lost just over a stone when he was born, so you can imagine what I
was like . . . and I just got that, you know, I don't care if the milk runs
out – I wanted to breast feed him but it got to the stage when it was

wrong for the marriage. I mean Alex couldn't stand the sight of me – I was wearing maternity dresses still and I thought 'I've got to do something about it.'

Clearly, pregnancy, breast feeding and looking after and feeding small children can produce changes in women's bodies which sometimes make it difficult for themselves and their partners to view their bodies as sexually attractive. But, equally clearly, women continue to want to achieve the unachievable – a pre-adolescent sylph-like shape – and this produces considerable conflict and guilt in their attitudes (and practices) towards food. Interestingly, almost the only time when it is acceptable for women to have a large body size is when they are pregnant and many women commented on this, remarking that it was the only time they were free from conflict and guilt over the food they ate. Perhaps this is one of the explanations for the indulgence of cravings during pregnancy, it is the *only* time in her life that a woman does not have to think of the effects of such indulgence on her shape:

I got inside my maternity dresses and I had a little more room to eat a bit more and I just went crackers I think. I had this nine months when it didn't really – I think I had it in the back of my mind that it didn't really matter – I'd put on a few pounds 'cos I'd got a bump at the front anyway and everybody knows I'm pregnant kind of thing.

However, women were often dismayed at what they saw as the price for this indulgence: 'I think any pregnant woman thinks "Well I'm fat anyway so I'll carry on eating." This was me anyway. It is stupid because it's very difficult to shift the weight afterwards. [She went from 10½ to 15 stones.] That was a terrible time.'

Many women found it much more difficult then to lose weight, usually precisely because of their changed circumstances and the fact that they are at home all day with temptation around. For most of the women we interviewed dieting was difficult (only 12 of those who were trying to diet said it was not) and for many it only became necessary after the birth of their first child or on marrying. A majority of them had given up work to look after their young children which meant that their days were not structured by any external factors. In addition they were, often for the first time, totally financially dependent on their partners. The three women quoted at the beginning of the chapter signified that these factors were important to them in creating problems in their relationship to food. For one, marriage and giving up work was linked to depression and turning to food for comfort. For another, the birth of her baby created stress and tension which caused her to turn to food for relief, and for the third, food belonged to her husband and her consumption of it signified her total dependence on him. She therefore denied herself any food over and above what she could buy with her child allowance which was, at the time, her only source of income.

This indicates that, along with the requirement of self-denial of food in the interests of sexual attraction or controlling a situation in which you are out of control (for instance in the third example above), indulgence in food is often a response to a stressful situation, and the life changes involved with giving up work and having children can clearly be extremely stressful. This resort to food as a relief from stress clearly makes self-denial doubly difficult. Thus, not only are women constantly surrounded by food and thinking about providing it for others, the stresses and tensions of their situation lead them to resort to food as a comfort. This, of course, produces guilt and more stress because a gain rather than the desired loss in weight may be the result. Women, therefore, find themselves in a vicious circle with food perceived as a friend and enemy at one and the same time.

Women deny themselves food in order to be slim and attractive but they *also* deny themselves food in order that their partners and children might eat adequately. Slimming can become a pretext for denying yourself food when money is tight and food is in short supply and it was fairly common amongst our sample for women to skip meals as part of a dieting strategy. The outcome of this seemed often to be that men and children ate while women hardly ate at all. The experience of one of the families dependent on supplementary benefit illustrates this point. In this family there were four children and two adults and the woman missed six main meals and six non-main meals during the two weeks that she filled in her food diary. She consumed far less than anyone else in the family and said that she was trying to lose weight. However, her comments when asked about taking her own likes and dislikes into consideration when planning meals indicate that this is not the whole story:

Well that doesn't matter 'cos I can go without anyway as long as I've got them sommat what they'd eat. I mean it's no good getting them sommat they're not going to eat even if it is cheap. [So you put yourself last, do you?] Yeah, well, *I* do. *He* likes to eat so we usually get something what he'd like.

Women, therefore, often practise self-denial for reasons other than the pursuance of the goal of slenderness, although this may be a not unwelcome outcome. What is significant about this self-denial, for whatever reason it is practised, is that women are denying themselves the pleasure that is associated with eating food; whether it be chocolates or cream cakes ('naughty but nice') or food presented in the form of a proper meal. Women, in other words, deny themselves pleasure, whereas one of their aims in preparing food for others is to give pleasure; women fundamentally cook to please men in particular. The denial of enjoyment, or the contradiction between enjoying food and the need to watch your weight, was brought out by one woman when talking about her daughter. She thought that she rather than her sons might have to reduce her food intake when she grew older:

I think Julia might later on. I think she'll have to be careful in her teens. Because she eats with gusto what is put in front of her and I think if she were given a free rein, if I were the sort of person who kept a lot of biscuits in the house, then she would be fat because she just enjoys eating.

And several women, while expressing dissatisfaction with their weight, did not actually do anything about it because they enjoyed their food 'too much'. Indeed, some women felt guilty about finding pleasure in food and felt that they were using food as a substitute for other forms of enjoyment. One woman linked her weight gain to the restrictions placed on her by having children:

It's just over the years [I've put on weight]. Well, having the children in one way, not because of having them but because it's cut out my social life and I – I think a lot of people are guilty of it – I turned food into a sort of pleasure and it's a bad habit.

This is interesting because it points to the different relationship to food experienced by women and men. Men can eat for pleasure and are expected to enjoy their food. Children, even, are given sweets and biscuits and puddings as treats, as a means of giving pleasure. And women see this as an important element of preparing food for others. But for themselves such enjoyment is somehow illicit, it induces guilt. Hence, the 'Naughty but Nice' slogan attached to adverts for cream. This captures the guilty pleasure associated with eating something that is forbidden – to women. And for some women enjoyment of food stood in the way of them dieting. The woman who turned to food in the stressful situation of having a small, demanding baby talked about this:

I enjoy eating, it gives me that satisfaction to relax and make me able to cope – I can't give it up really. I can talk to myself and say 'Don't be stupid, you don't want this', but still I go and get it. It's always biscuits and things like that – usually biscuits and that's all really because it's something to nibble at that you can just go and grab and eat.

In our culture it is particularly sweet foods which are associated with pleasure, and these were precisely those which were to be avoided by the would-be dieter. They are also the foods which are most commonly turned to as a source of comfort, and this is learned early on by children as we saw in Chapter 5. Thus, the lesson that food is a friend is learnt and internalised long before puberty and adolescence when food becomes an enemy to the sexually maturing young teenager.

Women often broke their diets, or allowed themselves to relax at certain times while they were dieting, and ate sweet foods of one sort or another. The pleasure and the guilt are brought out in the following comments:

I might spoil myself on a Sunday or if I'm feeling a bit low – with a chocolate bar or a piece of cake.

On a Sunday I eat normally and for six days I diet. I think you have to have something to look forward to.

Fresh cream cakes or other 'forbidden foods' might also be turned to as a comfort for not having lost weight: 'When I thought I've been particularly good for the last fortnight or whatever and I think "Oh, well, I should have lost five pounds" and I go on the scales and I still haven't lost anything, I think "Oh, to hell with it."' The woman who had almost stopped eating because of her dependence on her husband also went to a slimming club and, in common with many of the women, found it hard to stick to a diet without allowing herself to eat of the forbidden:

I went to slimming club. Me and my friend used to go to the slimming club on a Thursday night with about 90p. We used to come out of there, go to the pub and have some fish and chips on the way home and slim the rest of the week! I used to have me lax periods. That was my night out then, my husband never took me out. I went out three times in fifteen months. That was my night out, going to the slimming club, so I enjoyed it.

This sort of situation can become difficult to control, with indulgence in 'comfort' foods being compensated for by periods of strict dieting when no pleasure is derived from eating at all. In fact, there is some indication that self-control in the form of denying yourself food, denying one of the pleasures of the body, is a substitute for a lack of control of your social situation – although many women reacted differently and turned to food to comfort themselves in an unhappy situation. This was true of the woman who ate excessively due to depression whom we quoted at the beginning of the chapter. But it was also true in less extreme circumstances. One woman told us of her inability to control her biscuit consumption, an experience shared by many of the women.

I lived on Limmits for about two weeks to try to slim off a bit around April. I seemed to put on a bit of weight for no apparent reason. I do indulge myself in quite a lot of biscuits which I can't stop eating. I think it's because after I've done a lot of work or run around for the children or walked down to playgroup I suddenly feel ravenous when I come home and before I can do any work I have to sit down and eat something. [Oh, and once you start eating biscuits it's difficult to stop.] That's it, and I don't just have one, I mean I can sit down sometimes and it's like a meal – I eat half a packet before I can get up and do anything else. I've always done it, it's not something I suddenly started.

Self-control and self-denial are particularly difficult for women who are at home with young children all day because they are almost certainly going to be eating sweets and biscuits between meals, foods which could be kept out of the house entirely if children were not part of the household. One woman told us about her problems with dieting:

It's when other people are eating I think, when you're trying to cut down and you get that stage when you're feeling, not exactly starving, but you think you could just eat one of those sweets – that's when you want something that you can nibble. Really, it would be a lot better if you could eat something that was sweet – it's a craving for sweet things rather than anything else.

Many women shared this craving for sweet foods, particularly
when they were cutting down on their food intake, and several
of them mentioned that sweet foods were particularly hard to
resist in the week before their period. However, this craving was
not confined to that particular time in the menstrual cycle so it
clearly has social determinants whatever its physiological basis
may or may not be.

Dieting strategies

In the face of food consumption being a source of pleasure and a
comfort in times of stress, and the family situation which
requires women to provide food for men and children day in, day
out, how did women put into practice their desire to lose weight?
As we have seen, many women, although dissatisfied with their
bodies, did little or nothing in the way of reducing their food
intake. But 68 (34%) of the women were dieting or watching
their weight at the time of interview. The strategies they
adopted varied, but they were often a product of 'common sense';
very few women were following diets prescribed by health care
professionals. One woman's comments reveal the nature of the
common sense view of slimming and also point to the permanent
guilt there is about eating when women feel that they need to
lose weight. She was asked whether she was currently dieting or
had ever watched her weight:

No, not really. I mean I shouldn't have had a Chinese meal on Saturday
– I could have lived without it. No, it's sort of very half-hearted. [What
sort of food do you try to avoid, or is it more just cutting things down?]
Cutting things down I think. Probably not eating potatoes and cakes,
you know the things that I make for John and Timothy – just not have
any of those. [And do you try to eat any particular foods?] More fruit I
suppose, boring old fruit. It's not very satisfying . . . [Where do you get
your diet from?] Nowhere. Just what you hear people saying. I mean
there's a lady at [work] on a hard boiled egg and banana diet – she has it
every lunch time. But I don't take an awful lot of notice because if I
want to be really serious about it I know what I have to do deep down, I
mean we all do, don't we. Even really big ladies who need to lose
weight, they know in their heads what they've got to do to lose it, you
don't need to go to a doctor and get a diet sheet, all you need is will
power isn't it and the rest you know.

Dieting is a matter of common sense and will power according to
her, and most of the women agreed on the types of food which

should be avoided if a loss in weight was to be achieved – 37 (18·5%) mentioned bread and potatoes, 54 (27%) mentioned sweet foods and 21 (19·5%) mentioned fried foods. As we can see, sweet foods – foods which are regarded as pleasurable – come top of the list. This is interesting as they bear a striking similarity to the foods which were regarded as being 'bad' for you in general health terms.

It would seem, therefore, that concern over dieting and putting on weight to some extent informs women's views of healthy and unhealthy food. This was expressed by one woman who had regularly attended a slimming club and rigorously followed their diet:

It's a high protein, low carbohydrate diet that *I'm* on that helps as well when I'm planning meals for these lot. I think, 'Well, I'll give them more meat and veg. as opposed to a great plateful of mashed potato . . .' I'm thinking, 'Well, that wouldn't be good for me on the diet I'm following, so it can't be much good for them.'

This felt necessity to avoid bread and potatoes and sweet foods if women were dieting would clearly be problematic in the context of feeding a family. Bread and potatoes are staples of the British diet and potatoes are a constituent element of the proper meal. Sweet foods in the form of puddings are frequently given to children and are seen as appropriate for them, something they enjoy, while sweets and biscuits are eaten by children (and women) between meals, and cake, although consumed most frequently by men, is a pleasurable and desirable food. Women felt guilty, though, if their dieting meant that the rest of the family also had to go without these foods. 'Trev [husband] helps me by saying we can do without things like cakes, but then I don't think that's fair on him and the kids.' And this makes it hard for women to diet, the food that is prohibited is right under their noses being eaten and enjoyed by everyone else. 'Steve [husband] doesn't appreciate the sorts of things I'd eat while I'm dieting – like Ryvitas and salads. Makes it harder when he's getting potatoes and desserts and things.' Women were asked what dieting strategies they adopted and most frequently they cut down the amount of food they ate and, as we have already seen, avoided certain foods. Of the women 48 (24%) said they did this, 30 (15%) said they cut down on food and 17 (8·5%) said they avoided certain foods; 11 (5·5%) of the women said that they skipped meals altogether. Some women linked changes in weight with changes in their social circumstances. The woman who linked her weight gain to depression discussed the way she had finally lost weight:

I used to diet, yes. I used to attempt to diet at that time and I never found it particularly successful. I just found really through different changes in circumstances that my weight just seemed to gradually come down. It started coming down when we moved into a flat and we didn't have a proper cooker and I couldn't boil potatoes or make pies or anything else. I couldn't even heat things up properly with this oven, so we tended to eat a lot less then and without any conscious effort I just lost weight and then I worked in Leeds for so many months and living in York and I was working over and I didn't used to get in till ten at night and I lost weight then just 'cos I rushed around a lot. It's been circumstances that's made me lose it.

Clearly, however, she also restricts her intake of certain foods on a more or less permanent basis:

Well now I try and eat sensibly all the time so my weight doesn't go up. If I'm trying to cut down really I've gradually weaned myself completely off biscuits. I still have the odd ones here and there, I'm not completely anti-biscuits, you know, I mean not to offend somebody I would sometimes have one but I don't have biscuits. I don't really now not have anything at all really, I just try and eat a reasonable quantity of everything really.

We have already mentioned that significant life changes which may be stressful and which may result in a woman's loss of control over her own situation, such as leaving a job and becoming financially dependent on a man, can lead to food being used as a comfort. It can also, it seems, lead to women wanting to control their body size strictly and to do this they need to control their food intake. In this sense the obsession with food and the desire to lose 'just half a stone' or 'just a little bit more' before reaching the perfect shape or weight may be a product of women's lack of control in their daily lives. If they can control their bodies through strict control of their food intake perhaps the dissatisfactions that they experience would go. It is as if women's bodies are being blamed for their unsatisfactory social situation. And this may symbolically reflect a real situation, that women occupy a structurally different and less powerful position than men in our society, and the differentiating factor is our bodies. Reducing the size of our bodies, as Chernin and MacLeod have pointed out, is a way of minimising our differences, returning us to the relatively undifferentiated pre-pubertal state (Chernin, 1983; MacLeod, 1981). Anorexic women who cease to menstruate are on the way to achieving this and some of the women we spoke to had experienced amenorrhoea through the denial of food to their bodies. Several of the women also felt that they might easily become anorexic and that dieting and denying themselves food was in some way gratifying, in the words of one of the women: ' . . . depriving yourself is quite gratifying, it can be so, you feel very smug.'

Control over food intake was often precarious. In speaking of dieting strategies, one woman said:

If I don't want to eat, if I just have the one meal in the day then I'm fine. You see, when I worked I used to eat breakfast as well then but I didn't bother with lunch then, I just had an apple or something, but I was working all day, I wasn't really around food so that, you know, breakfast kept me going. Whereas now, if I've had breakfast I tend to think in the morning, 'I'd like a drink and a biscuit, now', or something, whereas if I don't have it, it doesn't set me off for some reason, it's weird, really.

And this was a common feeling. It also indicates how much more difficult this control is when women are at home all day with their enemy lurking in the kitchen waiting to catch them out at the first hint of weakness. This need to control the body and its relation to lack of control of the social situation was clear from one woman's experience. She felt that she could understand people who became anorexic. She said:

Whatever [weight] I am I always want to be less . . . I'm at my lowest weight that I've been for years at eight stone two pounds and yet I still feel I could do to lose a stone off . . . maybe it's to satisfy my own ego, I don't know. When I see thin women I admire them.

Before she married and had children she weighed ten stone two pounds.

When I was at work I was quite a confident person – maybe with going through all this – maybe I need to boost my confidence and maybe 'cos I'm at this weight maybe I keep thinking that if I could get half a stone off maybe I'd feel better, I don't really know.

She clearly feels that a weight reduction would ameliorate her stressful situation. Her husband had just left her with two small children (this is what she's referring to above) so her situation had recently changed dramatically and her lack of control and feelings almost of panic seem to be transferred on to a concern with her weight: 'At eight stone two pounds I feel that *I am in control* and that my clothes are OK. But it only takes a few pounds and then you sort of creep back up again to eight and a half, I panic a bit' (Our emphasis). Perhaps also women's almost obsessional concern over their food intake arises because it is the only area of their lives over which they are able to exercise total control. The woman who had been anorexic threw some light on this when she was asked whether her partner helped at all at mealtimes:

Well, he always volunteers and if there is anything I do want doing, he'll do it. But I'd rather he was out of the way, he's a bit clumsy. I think that's because I've been so locked up in the house for such a long time that it's got on top of me. I've been trying to explain it to him because we've had many an argument about it – I was trying to explain to him that when we first moved, upstairs was hoovered once a week and then it was getting more often. It got in the end it was every day, sometimes twice a day I was up there with the hoover. You see, the thing is it's because of having no outside interest, if there was something else I was interested in it wouldn't be too bad, but the only thing I *have* got is the home, so I concentrated too much on it. [Yes, it gets out of proportion.] Yes, and there's nothing you can do about it. I went on one of these slimming things, I must have been one of the first, it was before I was married . . . the obsession is just like that, like they've got this obsession not to eat, my obsession to go on with that hoover is exactly the same.

Such an obsession, involving rigid control over your food intake, is not easily maintained by most women, although it may be the desired goal. Most women's control over food was much more precarious. However, their problematic relationship to food, together with the dieting strategies they adopted, did not significantly affect the food intake of their partners and children. It was more usual that women's diets were jettisoned than that men and children were 'deprived' of puddings or potatoes. But this left women feeling constantly guilty, feeling that they *ought* to be dieting and *shouldn't* be eating biscuits or puddings, but as they were there and available they were unable to resist them. Partners' preferences in particular could scupper women's attempts to diet. The woman who felt she *ought* to diet but never quite got round to it told us that her husband 'goes nuts' about cakes and puddings which she considered were not an essential part of the family diet:

I came from a home where nobody had a sweet tooth at all and a cake would be there for a month and then you'd have to throw it away 'cos it was mouldy. But John has always been used to a pudding of some kind, so I started making things and then decided that if I ate it as well as him it would only be hanging around for two days instead of four, you see, that was my excuse.

It was very rare that men's weight was considered to be a problem in the same way as women's and that they would go on a diet together. So this mutual support was not available to women from their partners, although it sometimes was from friends who were also trying to diet. In fact, the family situation was constantly undermining women's diets. Often, if women ate something different from the rest of the family at mealtimes the children would insist that she share their food or that they share hers. And since the family meal is ideologically and practically important to women, it was again difficult for them to eat differently from the rest of their family. Hence the pursuit of slenderness and the ideal form of feminine sexual attractiveness came into grave conflict with the demands of motherhood *and* with the use of food as a comfort in times of stress. These contradictory demands on women, and the centrality of food (its provision or denial) to their conflicting roles, gives us some indication of why it is that women's relationship to food is so problematic within our culture.

Double standards

Concern over men's and children's weight was much less widespread and was much more frequently related to health or ill health than was the case for women. It is interesting to look at the family situation of the woman who had had a severe anorexic experience during her teens. She had a son and a daughter: her son was a very faddy eater whereas her daughter ate everything that was put in front of her. As a result, in their mother's eyes, he was skinny and she was fat:

Actually, sometimes I wish they were the other way round, I wish Robert had a bit more meat on him and Gemma was more like he is. I was saying to Bob, I know she has slimmed down an awful lot but when she was a baby I mean I used to say to Bob, 'Oh my, you know, a skinny boy and a big fat girl', but she has slimmed . . . [You think it wouldn't be so bad to have a tubby boy as a tubby girl?] I'd rather have neither, but if it was I'd rather the boy was than the girl was. [Why?] I don't know . . . little girls should be all nice, sweet little darlings, not big, fat, grotesque jobs.

She clearly reflects the different standards which are applied to boys and girls in relation to 'fatness'. Boys, as men, can get away with a lot more than girls. This differential standard is also clear when she speaks about her husband's weight:

He's five foot ten and I can't tell you exactly but he goes up and down somewhere in the region of thirteen and fourteen stone. He just can't lose it. It's not that he does eat a lot because specially for a man I suppose – if he has breakfast it's just a couple of slices of toast. If he has dinner it's just a sandwich and then he has a meal at night. I must admit I do pile it on and keep thinking 'Oh, he's the man, he should have a meal like that.'

Another woman was concerned about her partner's weight and her views are fairly typical:

I think he probably does eat too much fatty food. [What are you particularly worried about in that context?] Well, he is a bit over-weight, but I think the last medical he went for he was about ten pounds overweight, which isn't a great deal, it's enough but it isn't a great deal. But then again, he does get a lot of exercise, he is quite fit, he can run quite well and everything. But I still have this niggle about fatty foods and the heart.

This points to a difference between women's and men's relation to food. If men are living with women then usually the women cook for them, women regulate the amount of food that they provide for men – *and* for themselves. Men therefore do not directly control their own food intake in this context, food is given to them by someone else. Women, however, give food to themselves. In the context of cutting down on food it is interesting that women regarded it as *their* responsibility to 'cut their husbands down' if they were getting overweight. The men could undermine this, but it remains the case that men have someone looking after and worrying about their food intake; women do not once they no longer live at home with their mothers. Usually, though, if women felt men to have a weight problem it stemmed from a concern with the possibility of heart disease, or other health related issues, and men's dietary strategies usually involved taking more exercise rather than cutting down dramatically on food. But what is striking is that concern with men's weight was far less widespread than concern over women's. Almost half the men (90) were reported as never having dieted or expressed concern over their weight compared with only 23 of the 200 women. In addition, a dual standard was applied to men's and women's weight; men were allowed to be much heavier and larger than women relative to their size before they were deemed to have a weight problem.

Concern over children's weight, which was only expressed by a few women (11, 5·5%), was almost always linked to the social unacceptability of 'fat' children and the cruelty of their peers rather than health concerns. One woman felt herself to be a bit on the fat side and loved all types of sweet foods which she tried to keep away from. One of her daughters she thought might take after her:

I was a fat child – I hated it. I mean I'm not thin now, but as you get older you can cope with it, but as a child I don't want her to be fat and I don't want her to be picked on because she's fat. I don't mind her being plump but I don't want her to be fat, so I tend to sort of watch her, what she's eating. Not Tracey . . . she can eat more or less anything, she doesn't put on any weight.

She said that her other daughter was as skinny as a rake but had already become aware of the possibility of becoming fat:

. . . even Tracey [3½ years] has been watching Grange Hill, and there's been a thing on Grange Hill about a little boy who's very fat, and it quite upset Tracey did this, 'I don't want to be fat when I go to school' and 'I'm not going to overeat and make myself fat 'cos I don't want them laughing at me at school.' Well – it's brought into them from a young age that it's the thing to be slim, well I mean she's no worry at all, I said to her 'You can keep on eating for ever more.'

Women therefore not only monitor their own weight but are concerned over their partners and children. But it seems that this concern takes a different form. For children concern arises in case they are made fun of at school, for men it is likely to be because of the fear of ill-health arising from obesity, but for women themselves, it is a concern to achieve a sylph-like sexually alluring body. This aim sits ill with the physically

demanding tasks associated with child rearing and housework.
One woman had been dieting and told us:

Well, I tried to lose a bit but I find that it doesn't suit me. I get tired. I
went down to eight stone after I had David and I felt real drawn. I went
back – no I like to stay just under eight and a half stone, I feel well at
that. I'd like to be a bit thinner but I'm happy at that and I can manage
whereas when I was a bit less I seemed to be a bit drawn and tired
looking.

Dieting can leave a woman without the strength to be the
ideal mother and housewife, although she might in this manner
attain the shape to be the ideal lover. This contradiction was
experienced by the majority of women we spoke to and involves
them in a never ending 'battle of the bulge', something which is
not experienced by men and which makes women's relationship
to food particularly contradictory and problematic.

8

Class and food provision

In the preceding chapters we have concentrated on women's relationship to food within the family and we have described the way family food practices mark and reinforce social divisions of gender and age. We have argued that practices at this level of daily life actively reinforce unequal relations of power and status within the family. In this and the following chapter we turn our attention to the ways in which families differ from each other in the food they eat and the way they eat it. We shall concentrate specifically on class differences between families which exist despite the powerful unifying presence of family ideology. We shall also explore the ways in which gender divisions and relations between parents and children are mediated by occupational class. The specific areas which we focus on are daily food provision, the use of food in hospitality and entertaining and patterns of food consumption.

Food ideologies and income

Perhaps the three most important variables which influence family food practices and which are themselves linked to class are income, hours of work and food ideologies. The first two are self-explanatory but the third deserves some elaboration. Food ideology refers to sets of beliefs and attitudes which inform food practices. Julia Twigg has analysed vegetarianism as a food ideology, which she counterposes to the dominant food ideology (Twigg, 1983). Within this dominant food ideology meat is the most highly valued food, other animal products are less highly valued and vegetables, cereals and pulses come at the bottom of the food hierarchy. So within this ideology meat is afforded a central place and its consumption is regarded as essential. This food ideology informs the way most of the women we spoke to think about food. The central element of the 'proper meal' is meat and families' diets are structured around its provision in this form. Vegetarian food ideologies, however, embrace different value systems. Meat is not highly valued, indeed it is not eaten at all, and foods which are not valued in terms of the dominant food ideology, such as beans and pulses occupy a central place. Vegetarianism often goes hand in hand with a political critique of the world food system, which argues that meat production is an expensive and wasteful use of resources, and that the world food problem would be soluble if meat was eaten less often in the advanced industrialised countries, so freeing more resources for the production of cereals and vegetables. The adoption of an 'alternative' food ideology can, therefore, be a protest. As Kim Chernin (1986) has pointed out it can mark a daughter's assertion of independence and we would extend this to argue that it can also involve an attempt to distance yourself from, not only the dominant food ideology, but also other dominant ideologies, such as family ideology, of which the proper meal of meat and two veg is such an important part. Food can therefore be part of an 'alternative' lifestyle, a way of living that attempts to distance itself from dominant attitudes and values. Conversely, acceptance of these attitudes and values involves an adherence to food practices which are culturally and ideologically appropriate to the family. It was only a small minority of the women we spoke to who articulated alternative food ideologies and they were almost totally confined to occupational classes I/II. Significantly one of these women was living on state benefit and her diet was markedly different from the other families on state benefit. (See Charles and Kerr (1968a) for a more detailed discussion of this point.) This indicates that income alone cannot account for differences in diet; ideologies and cultural values are also important.

However, for families whose diets are constructed within the dominant food ideology, and they constituted the majority of our sample, income plays a large part in determining the food they eat. Thus, although most women felt proper meals were essential for family eating, their ability to provide food in this form depended to a large extent on their income, or the income of their partners. Families' incomes were closely correlated to men's occupational class, which is clearly what would be expected given that the occupational hierarchy is differentiated by differences in pay – the higher up the hierarchy the higher the financial reward – and that most of the women were not working in paid employment. As we can see from Table 8.1, high earnings were confined to men in classes I and II (with one exception) and non-manual workers were much more likely to earn a middle level of income than manual workers. Low earners were typically manual workers and were most likely to be in classes IV and V, while male unemployment amongst our sample was confined to manual workers.

Daily food provision

It seems that class profoundly influences the way women experience the tasks that are assigned to them and the options that are open to them in terms of providing food for their families, and that one of the major ways it does this is through its effect on income. Perhaps shopping for food is the most obvious point at which to begin our discussion of daily food provision as the amount of money coming into a household directly affects what can and cannot be bought.

We have already pointed out that in the majority of families it is women who decide what food to buy and it is interesting to look at the effect of class on the factors they take into account when considering what food to prepare for their families. Family food preferences were cited as the most important consideration by most of the women closely followed by the 'goodness' of food and its cost. It was also thought important that food should be fresh although few women thought that it was important to emphasise filling the family up, the time taken to prepare meals and the appearance of food. What really came through in the women's responses to this question, though, was the variability in the process of food preparation and the extent to which the factor given the most importance depends on what has happened during the day. This meant that quantifying the women's responses became very difficult and imposed a rather artificial order on a process that was dynamic and dependent on

Table 8.1 Income level of family by occupational class of men (n = 197 – no. (%) excluding the family where the partner is in gaol and students)

	I/II	IIIN	IIIM	IV/V	Single parent	Total
Unemployed/single parent	–	–	5 (6)	1 (5·0)	10 (100)	16 (8)
Low income (less than £80/week)	1 (2)	2 (7)	10 (13)	7 (33·0)	–	20 (10)
Low/middle income (£80–£100/week)	8 (13)	9 (32)	34 (44)	5 (24·0)	–	56 (28)
Middle income (over £100/week – Less than £10,000 per year)	34 (57)	10 (36)	12 (15)	2 (9·5)	–	58 (29)
High income (over £10,000/year)	10 (17)	1 (4)	–	–	–	11 (6)
Don't know	6 (10)	4 (14)	13 (17)	4 (19·0)	–	27 (14)
Other/missing	1 (2)	2 (7)	4 (5)	2 (9·5)	–	9 (5)
Total	60 (100)	28 (100)	78 (100)	21 (100·0)	10 (100)	197 (100)

Table 8.2 Frequency of food shopping by occupational class of male partner – no. (%)

	I/II	IIIN	IIIM	IV/V	Single parent	Total
Daily	6 (10)	4 (14)	6 (8)	3 (14)	2 (20)	21 (10·5)
Several times a week	6 (10)	4 (14)	10 (13)	2 (10)	4 (40)	26 (13·0)
Once a week	24 (40)	12 (43)	49 (63)	14 (67)	4 (40)	106 (53·0)
Less than once a week	23 (38)	6 (21)	13 (17)	2 (10)	–	44 (22·0)
Not given	1 (2)	2 (7)	–	–	–	3 (1·5)
Total	60 (100)	28 (100)	78 (100)	21 (100)	10 (100)	200 (100·0)

changing circumstances. One of the women's comments illustrates this well.

Well it depends on certain days, you see. It says 'time taken in preparation', well there's certain days that I don't mind preparing for them and other days when I can't be bothered. It's sometimes important and sometimes it's not. Sometimes I haven't got time to make a meal that needs a lot of preparation and there's some days when I'll say 'I'll do this' even if it takes a while . . . They are all important, they all are in a way, you see. It's like I say I don't worry about food that's good for you but I must put a certain amount of thought into it . . . I like fresh food and it's no good giving them anything that's not going to fill them. The cost is very important. I don't think the time taken in preparation is important as I say because day by day I feel different about that. Some days I don't particularly want to cook a meal, I don't feel like it.

Despite these difficulties it did seem that class affected the way these factors interacted in decision-making about food. Thus, women in social classes I/II were more likely than others to attach a high priority to the goodness of food, while women in classes IV and V were more likely to put the cost of food as their first consideration. For instance, 33% of women in social classes I/II placed 'food that is good for you' first in their list of priorities when considering what to make for a meal and 31% of them put it second; no women in social classes IV/V put it first. Conversely 33% of social class IV/V women placed cost first compared with 17% of women in classes I/II, 16% of women in class IIIN and 17% of women in class IIIM. Occupational class therefore, at least partly because of its links with level of income, constrains women in their decision-making about the food they buy. Women who have to count every penny have less opportunity than women who are relatively comfortably off to concern themselves with issues of goodness; they are constrained to buy what they can afford to ensure that their families eat 'properly'.

The constraints of income and class were also evident in the women's shopping patterns. Most women shopped at supermarkets for their 'main' shop and then used specialist shops such as butchers and greengrocers for fresh foods. A lot of women commented that going to buy bread or something for lunch at the local shop gave them a reason to get out of the house; it was regarded as a welcome break, an outing. One woman said:

It's a trip out and you take the baby for a walk. I might even go once a day, just to even buy a loaf of bread. It seems a silly thing to do but unless I'm going somewhere – I have to get somewhere to go – and unless you go to your friends for coffee, well, you do your housework and you think 'Now what can I do?'. It's an excuse 'I must pay my paper bill' or I reason it out in the week just to go out.

However, very few women shopped only at local shops. Even those with no means of transport and little money to pay bus fares managed to get to the supermarket for their main shop; and for some this meant a two or three mile walk with a pram and a toddler. Most of the women (104 – 52%) used a combination of local shops and a supermarket for food shopping and a further 69 (34·5%) used these in combination with the market. Eleven (5·5%) of the women used only local shops, 9 (4·5%) used a supermarket only, 3 used local shops and the market and 4 used a supermarket and the market. This pattern was not affected by social class but what *was* affected was the frequency of the main shop, or whether one took place at all, the use of wholefood shops, and who actually shopped for food.

The frequency of food shopping is related to men's occupational class in Table 8.2. As we can see, only a minority of women indulged in daily shopping although single parents seem rather more likely to than other women. Similarly shopping more than once a week was fairly evenly spread across the classes, again with the exception of single parents. Shopping once a week, however, was more likely to be the pattern of women whose partners were in occupational classes IIIM, IV and V then those whose partners were in occupational classes I, II and IIIN, and shopping less than once a week shows a clear class gradient, with women whose partners were in classes I/II much more likely than other women to shop on perhaps a fortnightly or monthly basis. It is, of course, easier to do a large monthly shop if women drive a car or have access to one and if they have enough money to cover such a large outlay at one time. They also need storage facilities such as freezers and fridges. Four of the women we talked to did not have fridges: three of these were living on state benefits and the other was on a low income. Two of them shopped daily and the others shopped once a week. Another clear difference that emerged was in bulk buying. Meat for the freezer and, less commonly, groceries and vegetables were bought in bulk by some of the women. The breakdown of these figures shows a clear class correlation with 48% of women in classes I and II doing some bulk buying compared with 39% of women in occupational group IIIN, 27% of women in occupational group IIIM and 24% of women in classes IV/V. This again reflects possession of storage facilities and transport. Clearly these factors are all related to income, for most of our families to the man's income, therefore to his occupational class.

Another factor differentiating families from one another and affecting the frequency of shopping and what could be bought was the way in which the wage or salary was paid: whether money came into the household weekly, fortnightly (as in the case of social security and unemployment benefit), monthly, or even less frequently, as with student grants and ministers' stipends. It was usual for the lower income families to be dependent on a weekly wage or fortnightly benefit and this in itself made it difficult to undertake a monthly shop. Budgeting was usually planned on a weekly basis, certain sums being put by for bills and the rest being spent on food and other necessities. One woman, managing on her partner's unemployment benefit, described the juggling exercise that had to be performed every fortnight.

It depends how much you've spent on your bills that week as to what you've got left for your food . . . If it's tele week then that's £10.75 and say you've missed an insurance the week before so you've got two lots of insurance to pay and you're left with next to nowt. I mean I've known times when we've had pie and chips for Sunday dinner instead of a proper Sunday dinner.

Women whose partners were on low incomes also had to count every penny. A woman whose husband earned £65 a week said: 'Well first of all we sort out all the bills when he brings home his wages and whatever's left out of his wages I get the tinned stuff. When I get my family allowance on a Monday that goes on meat and things like that for the week.' This comment underlines the importance of child benefit (family allowance) for families on low incomes; it is essential to enable the family to eat. Often, however, families dependent on state benefits could not make the money stretch to cover food for the week or fortnight, and their experiences bring home to us why the cost of food far outweighs other considerations when deciding on what food to prepare for themselves and their families. One woman whose partner was unemployed said:

I mean sometimes we used to have nothing at all in the house and I used to go rushing down to my mam's saying 'Can we come for dinner 'cos I've only got enough left in for my tea' and you know 'We don't get paid till morning'. It's usually the last two days before you get your pay that you've got next to nowt in. Now I always get stuff off the milkman (on tick) so that's not so bad.

This woman's experience shows how important the extended family, particularly mothers and sisters, can be in reducing food costs for families with very low incomes. But it also shows how easy it is for these families to get into debt. While many women coped by putting aside money for constant outgoings such as bills before spending anything on food, others felt that food was of prime importance and the rest would take care of itself. As one woman in a low income family said:

If you eat right and well it doesn't matter about the other things I don't think. Like gas bill if it comes and I think oh chuck it, if I haven't got it they can't squeeze it out of me, you know just wait until we get the red letter or until we can afford it, something's bound to turn up and luckily up to now it has you know.

However, despite this privileging of food, most women on low incomes did not feel that they could feed their families in the way that they would like to. We asked all the women if they could buy all the food that they would like to buy. Many women in this context mentioned 'luxury' foods, food that they would buy as a treat but which they did not regard as being an essential part of the diet. Included here were foods such as lobster, caviar, gateaux, etc., foods which they did not normally buy. But others felt they were unable to buy foods that should be a part of daily eating and this was, unsurprisingly, related to their level of income. Only 12% of the families dependent on state benefits felt they could afford all the food they would like to buy compared with 30% of women in low income families, 43% of women in low/middle income families, 41% of women in middle income families and 72% of women in high income families. Here it is important to bear in mind that within the dominant food ideology foods are hierarchically ranked and those with the highest social value are also those that cost the most. Additionally the proper meal was regarded as central to a family diet. Women managing on low incomes most often expressed their inability to feed their families 'properly' in terms of the provision of a proper meal containing meat of a relatively high social status. Other foods which women on low incomes felt unable to afford were cakes, biscuits, fresh fruit, fresh vege- tables and butter. Indeed, it could be argued that the importance of meat in the diet, and the necessity to include it in the proper meal, contributed to their inability to buy other foods, precisely because meat is expensive. And particularly expensive is the Sunday joint, a meal which most women went to great lengths to preserve. It, together with the proper meal, holds symbolic as well as nutritional significance for the preservation of the family.

While women on higher incomes regretted the higher cost of entertaining with food, those managing on less money usually talked to us about the difficulties of providing 'good' meat for their families. Indeed many of them felt that because they had to resort to cheese or eggs, or 'improper' meat, such as sausages and beefburgers, they were not managing to feed their families properly. And by this, of course, they meant that they were unable to provide a 'cooked dinner' regularly and a Sunday 'dinner' at the weekend. Almost without exception their values were those of the dominant food ideology. Within this ideology an acceptable diet for a family is closely defined and any deviation from it reflects on the nature of that family. Indeed Sunday 'dinner' held a great significance and it was often the only meal which remained proper. Many women made stren- uous budgeting efforts throughout the week in order to ensure its status even in a diminished form. One woman whose husband earned a low income said:

I think we get enough nutritional value out of what we're eating but I don't think we ever eat properly. I class eating properly as a meal every night or a cheesey meal, sommat like that, a big meal every night but we just can't afford it. Our piece of beef that we have on a Sunday and we probably would have a cheese pie on a Tuesday and fish meal we'll probably have tonight. I do that type of routine and on other nights they usually have tinned things like meat balls.

Another woman whose husband was unemployed said:

We don't eat a lot of meat . . . they have a good amount of bread and that's good for energy for you. I know potatoes are not very good for you but they like chips so I mean – when he's out of work you can't really balance it if it isn't the right food. You've got to give them the ones that are sort of cheap and there's not much that's really good for you . . . the only day we eat properly is on a Sunday – Sunday's is the only big meal that we have. We have the chicken and new potatoes and cauliflower or cabbage.

The importance of preserving proper meal consumption in some form, even if it was less frequent and of lower status, ran through all the comments of women managing on low incomes and most of them felt that as long as a cooked dinner could be provided daily they were eating properly and adequately, although not as well as they would like. One woman whose partner was unemployed said she'd like to buy 'silverside for a weekend',

But there again – I mean I say this but I mean if you do brisket right you've got a lovely meal just the same. I think it's just the thought actually of what you can't afford that makes you want it rather than the actual need for it. I mean I think as long as you get a good square dinner in front of them every day they can't go far wrong.

However, many women felt themselves unable to do precisely this. Low incomes meant that the regular provision of proper meals became problematic, cheaper meats had to be resorted to and other foods were not bought at all. The preservation of the proper meal was felt to be crucial, not only to ensure that the family was eating properly but also to maintain it as a proper family. As we have already pointed out, the values placed on foods are influenced by food ideologies. These ideologies, therefore, affect the impact of income on a family's diet. Most of the women managing on low incomes adhered to the dominant food ideology in which meat occupies a central place. There was, however, one woman living on state benefits who adopted an 'alternative', mainly vegetarian diet and she was the only one who felt that she was able to eat a healthy diet on such a low income. In addition, she was able to buy foods that other women on low incomes were not. She was even able to buy alcohol, something that most women in low income families did not see from one year's end to the next. Importantly, as well as being the only woman on a low income to espouse an 'alternative' food ideology, she was also the only one from social class I or II. These two factors are not unrelated as 'alternative' food ideologies are more likely to be found amongst women in social classes I and II than in other social classes. Class, therefore, as well as largely determining income, also affects food ideologies; and the interaction of the two rather than income alone has to be taken into account when assessing the impact of income on families' diets. Having said that, however, almost all the women in our sample felt that the meat was a central component of a 'proper' diet and income clearly affected their ability to feed their families 'properly'. Additionally, the experience of low income was largely confined to women whose partners were unskilled manual workers and, less often in our sample, skilled manual workers; precisely those who are least likely to espouse an 'alternative' food ideology.

Given the prevalence of these attitudes, and almost all the women's concern to provide proper meals regularly for their partners and children, the experience of women in working-class families, particularly those on low incomes, was very different from those in middle-class homes who were comfortably off. The former had to constantly struggle to provide proper meals, and were often unable to do so. The latter were able to do so without worrying about the money at all. This difference, we suggest, clarifies the seeming lack of importance attached to nutritional issues among working-class women; it is not that they are not concerned to feed their families properly, it is that they have other worries and concerns which have to take precedence. This may also help to explain why there are differences according to women's class in the use of smaller, 'specialist' shops such as bakers and greengrocers, as opposed to the large and cost-saving supermarket. As we can see in Table 8.3 women in class IV/V are rather less likely than others to go to butchers, bakers and, particularly, wholefood shops. The class variation in the use of wholefood shops is particularly interesting as it reflects the greater concern with the 'goodness' of food characteristic of women in occupational classes I/II, and perhaps partly explains the middle-class image that these types of shops have which can make working-class people reluctant to go into them. We have correlated such patterns with women's own occupational class because we found that, as with women's attitude towards health and diet, such refinements of emphasis (whether women pay some attention to recent nutritional

Table 8.3   *Use of certain shops by women's occupational class – no. (%)*

	Butcher		Baker		Greengrocer		Wholefood shop	
I/II	29	(69)	18	(43)	39	(93)	13	(31)
IIIN	76	(73)	28	(27)	82	(79)	3	(3)
IIIM	20	(69)	7	(24)	20	(69)	1	(3)
IV/V	9	(50)	3	(17)	13	(72)	–	–
Total	134	(67)	56	(28)	154	(77)	17	(8·5)

advice, whether they patronise wholefood shops, prefer to buy their vegetables and bread fresh and so on) are more clearly related to women's class than the class of their partners. However, the material circumstances which constrain food provision, particularly income level, are, as we have already shown, more closely related to men's occupational class.

In Chapter 3 we noted that the majority of families operated a fairly rigid division of labour according to gender with women generally doing all, or at least most, of the cooking, shopping and other tasks surrounding food provision. But as we can see in Tables 8.4 and 8.5 the extent to which men helped with these tasks on a regular or irregular basis varied according to their occupational class. Although the class pattern varies somewhat according to whether it is shopping or cooking which is highlighted, it is clear that men in classes I and II were much more likely to help out with these tasks than their working-class counterparts. Involvement in shopping was particularly low for men in classes IV and V and as far as cooking was concerned it seems that skilled manual workers (those in class IIIM) were least likely to prepare meals. Similar contrasts between middle-class and working-class men were found when we looked at men's help with the subsidiary tasks of washing up and laying and clearing the table. What is interesting about these figures is that they indicate that the form taken by the gender division of labour varies with social class. This is reflected in middle-class men's seemingly greater willingness to participate in these domestic tasks. It is also apparent in the variation in patterns of money management where, although a housekeeping system with the man giving the woman a set amount of money each week or month is the most common arrangement, a joint system

Table 8.4 *Responsibility for meal preparation by social class of male partner – no. (%)*

	I/II	IIIN	IIIM	IV/V	Student	No partner	Total
Self prepares all meals	32 (53·3)	16 (57·1)	52 (66·7)	13 (61·9)	1 (50)	6 (60)	120 (60·3)
Self mainly, partner sometimes	24 (40·0)	9 (32·1)	16 (20·5)	7 (33·3)	–	–	56 (28·1)
Either or both (50/50)	–	–	1 (1·3)	1 (4·8)	–	–	2 (1·0)
Self mainly with help from partner and/or children sometimes	–	3 (10·7)	6 (7·7)	–	–	2 (20)	11 (5·5)
Other	4 (6·7)	–	3 (3·8)	–	1 (50)	2 (20)	10 (5·0)
Total	60 (100·0)	28 (100·0)	78 (100·0)	21 (100·0)	2 (100)	10 (100)	199 (100·0)

Table 8.5 *Food shopping – participants by occupational class of partner (n = 197) – no. (%)*

	I/II	IIIN	IIIM	IV/V	Single parent	Total
Women alone	18 (30)	14 (50)	35 (45)	15 (71)	10 (100)	92 (46·7)
Women with some help from partner	30 (50)	12 (43)	34 (44)	6 (29)	–	82 (41·6)
Women and/or partner	11 (18)	2 (7)	7 (9)	–	–	20 (10·2)
Partner only	1 (2)	–	2 (3)	–	–	3 (1·5)
Total	60 (100)	28 (100)	78 (100)	21 (100)	10 (100)	197 (100·0)

of money management is more common amongst class I/II households than those in the other social classes. This is discussed in detail in Kerr and Charles (1986). However, it has to be stressed that, despite this, in the majority of families women are the ones who shoulder the main burden of domestic tasks.

Meal organisation

Class not only influenced the type of food that could be bought by families and the gender division of labour around food provision, it also affected the way meals were organised and what foods were eaten by whom. In the rest of this chapter we concentrate on the effects of class on the organisation of daily eating and, in the next chapter, move to a discussion of the food that is actually consumed by families.

Most of the families we spoke to ate three meals a day, one of which was (ideally) a proper meal. On a Saturday meals tended to be more flexible and many women reported that they 'didn't really cook', whereas on a Sunday a Sunday 'dinner' was eaten, usually at midday, and many families also ate a cooked breakfast. There are, however, gender and age differences in the number of meals eaten. This is shown in Table 8.6. For instance on weekdays, apart from 17 families whose meal pattern was irregular, there were only two families in which the children ate less than three meals a day. However, the number of adults eating less than three meals a day was much higher and included more women than men. Thus in 36 families men regularly ate less than three meals a day but in 48 families women ate less. The figures for Saturdays and Sundays show a similar pattern with more women eating less than three meals a day than men, and almost all children eating three meals daily.

Table 8.6 also shows that although a majority of families eat three meals a day families of unemployed men are less likely to do so than others. Additionally, a lower proportion of single-parent households and families in occupational groups III, IV and V eat three meals a day than do families in classes I, II and IIIN. We would argue that these differences are probably due to income levels. This can be seen particularly clearly in the families of unemployed men where children usually eat three meals but adults may eat one or two meals daily. This was also

Table 8.6 *Partner's class by number of meals eaten on weekdays – no. (%)*

	I/II	IIIN	IIIM	IV/V	Single parent	Unemployed	No information	Total
All eat three	44 (73)	23 (82)	45 (62)	12 (60)	6 (60)	2 (33)	3 (100)	135 (67·5)
All eat two	–	–	2 (3)	–	–	–	–	2 (1·0)
Partner and children eat three, self one or two	6 (10)	–	5 (7)	1 (5)	–	–	–	12 (6·0)
Children eat three, partner two, self one or two	3 (5)	2 (7)	9 (12)	1 (5)	–	3 (50)	–	18 (9·0)
Children eat three, self and partner vary	6 (10)	2 (7)	6 (8)	2 (10)	–	–	–	16 (8·0)
Varies/other	1 (2)	1 (4)	6 (8)	4 (20)	4 (40)	1 (17)	–	17 (8·5)
Total	60 (100)	28 (100)	73 (100)	20 (100)	10 (100)	6 (100)	3 (100)	200 (100·0)

the case in four of the single-parent households but only happened in a minority of other families. It is also interesting that women denying themselves food in the form of missing meals, to a greater extent than men, occurs throughout the class structure and is not limited to families on low incomes. It is also not limited to women who are currently dieting. Interestingly in families where men were unemployed both the adults reduced their food intake while maintaining that of their children. In single-parent households, on the other hand, more women were able to eat three meals a day. This suggests that women's self-denial might be more frequent in families with men present, and that it may relate to men's supposed need to eat meat.

The timing of meals

The three meals eaten by families were breakfast, a main meal and a non-main meal. If a meal was missed it was often breakfast (although this was considered an important meal for children it was not for adults) and, less often, the non-main meal. The main meal was hardly ever missed. Few families ate a fourth meal in the evening and men were more likely to do so than anyone else. (In 106 households men ate a fourth meal at weekends. This was true for women in 77 of the households and children in 36. In 83 families a fourth meal was not eaten by anyone.) The timing of the main meal depended on when everyone could be at home to eat, and in families with young children this usually depended on the man's hours of work. In some households men were able to come home at midday and the main meal would be eaten then. In most however, men were out at work all day, older children were at school, and the only time the family could eat together was in the evening. On weekdays 143 (71·5%) of the families ate the main meal in the evening, 11 (5·5%) ate it at midday and 24 (12%) varied; in 16 of the families the adults ate in the evening while the children ate at midday. This practice was almost totally confined to social class I/II families. There was very little class variation in this pattern, but among the 24 families who varied their mealtimes there were 14 in which the men worked shifts. In order for the main meal to be eaten together its timing depended on the shift pattern of the men. The weeks they were on 6 to 2, for instance, the main meal was in the early evening;

when they were on 2 to 10, it was midday. One woman explained how it worked in her household:

Well it depends what shift John's working you see. When he's on the night shift or the morning shift then we always have our main meal at teatime. And when he's on the afternoon shift he's at work so we have our main meal at lunchtime, it's always when he's home. And then me and Tracey just have more of a snack really when we're on our own.

The unusual (in our sample) situation of shifts highlights the importance of men's hours of work for determining the timing of the main meal. The more usual situation is described by another woman:

I always want one good meal every day so I organise the main meal for teatime so that my husband can come in and enjoy it because he likes to be with the children. He certainly doesn't like to miss seeing them because some mornings he rarely sees much of them anyway. Usually he sees them to say hello and give them a kiss before he goes to work but I think the evening meal is the only one we all have in common so I make it the main meal . . . I mean I might be lazy but I just can't face cooking two meals a day. I'm the one who does the washing up and one big meal a day is enough to wash up for. As I say we get by until teatime.

Another important consideration was the need to get children bathed and into bed and not to make them wait too long for their main meal. In households where men finished work at 4 p.m. the main meal could be out of the way by 5.30 p.m. or 6 p.m., in plenty of time for the children to go to bed. However, where men did not finish work until 5 p.m. or even later the timing of the meal could be problematic. Most women were not keen on feeding the children earlier as it would have meant them cooking twice. Some, however, fed the children at midday and then ate with their partners later in the evening and one or two ate with the children at midday then cooked separately for their partners in the evening. In most families the evening meal during the week was served as soon as the man got in from work, but this was determined not only by his hours of work but also by the tiredness of the children. Women commented on the problems of organising meals with so many conflicting considerations. One woman, when asked if she enjoyed cooking, spoke about the difficulties of cooking a meal when the children were hungry and tired.

You see it's very difficult now with her because I don't enjoy a lot of things with her now. I enjoy her but teatime – she goes to bed, as I say, at 6, so at half past 4 or 5 o'clock I'm cooking tea and if my husband's not in she wants – I did have a tendency to give her biscuits to shut her up and she knows it's teatime and she's hungry and she's up my legs and I'm glad to get it (cooking) over with now.

Hardly any women responded to this by staggering meal times except for the 16 who fed their children their main meal at midday and themselves ate in the evening. Another way round this problem was for men to eat their main meal at midday at work, the women and children ate theirs at home also at midday and the evening was left free. This strategy was only adopted by a few women, most felt it important that all the family eat together at least once during the day and much effort was expended to ensure this happened.

In fact on weekdays 124 families ate their main meal together, on a Saturday 142 families ate it together and on a Sunday 162. However, class I/II families seemed less likely to eat together than families in other occupational classes during the week, although it was still a majority that did so. On Saturdays and Sundays this difference disappeared. (53% of class I/II families ate their main meal together on a weekday compared with 68% of class IIIN, 65% of IIIM and 62% of classes IV/V. On a Saturday, the figures are 73% of classes I/II, 57% of class IIIN, 69% of class IIIM and 71% of class IV/V, and on a Sunday they are 77% of I/II, 78·6% of IIIN, 83% of IIIM and 62% of IV and V. This is according to men's social class.) One of the women in a middle-class family described their eating pattern. She had two daughters, one aged 4½ and one aged 1½, and she and her partner were both working full time.

I prefer the children to have their main meal at lunch time because they get noticeably tired when they're hungry and it seems to re-fuel them in the middle of the day. They have a light breakfast so they seem to want to have more then so it seems appropriate to spread the load over the day. The reason why my husband and I don't have our main meal at lunch time during the week and then say have a high tea when we come home is that I find that if I eat a lot in the middle of the day it makes me very sleepy ... my husband is often working flat out in the middle of the day.

She envisaged the whole family eating together in the evening when the children were older. On Sundays, when they were all at home, they had their main meal together at midday. 'My husband and I will tend to have a proper lunch with the children instead of having the usual sandwich or whatever we have at work so we don't need a cooked meal in the evening.' The sorts of factors governing the timing of meals are illuminated in the following discussion between ourselves and one of the women.

[Can you tell me why you organise your meals like this?] Not many people do come home for lunch now do they? [I don't know, it's surprising how many I've come across who do and they always say 'I bet nobody else does'.] Because I said to him about the heating costs in the winter because he leaves me the car you see and he has a Honda and he goes on that. Of course when he gets home at lunch time he's freezing and of course when you sit down for a meal in there it's cold if I haven't got the heating on. He'll say 'put the heating on for me coming home' you know, and I'll say to him 'well look', I says, 'there's an answer now to it all, *they* can stop packed lunch, you stop at work with some sandwiches and I'll sit round the fire with my sandwiches and we'll have a meal on a night.' 'Oh no,' he says, 'I'm coming home.' It breaks his day up you see and of course James thinks it's awful because every other child in the class stops packed lunch and he wants to stop packed lunch. Well Alan got to that phase so I let him stop a couple of times and I think he found out that it wasn't as great as what he thought it was, it was a long day so he doesn't mind coming home. [So will you let James do that?] I'll maybe let him get it out of his system. [So it's really 'cos your husband likes . . .] It's my husband coming home and he has to be back for 1.45 you see. The kids get here at 12.20 and by the time I've cooked what I'm cooking it's 12.40 so it's more or less timed. I have the tea ready for them at 4.10. [So it's really his hours of work?] Mm.

Eating the main meal at midday was an uncommon practice generally; only 15 families in the whole sample did this. Additionally there was some irregularity in the timing of the main meal in occupational classes IV/V and amongst families of unemployed men, but most (145) families, no matter what their class, ate their main meal in the evening as a family.

Eating at Table

Even though in most families meals were eaten together there was a considerable variation in exactly what form the to-getherness took! For instance, some families always ate the main meal of the day at table while in others it was eaten in the sitting room in front of the television. In still others the women and children might eat at table without the television while men had their meal on a tray in an easy chair watching television.

A majority of families ate their meals at table. For instance the main meal on a weekday was eaten at table in 147 of the households; this figure increased to 167 for the main meal on Sunday. However, there seemed to be a distinction between adults and children, with children being more likely to eat at table than adults; this was true of all meals both during the week and at weekends. We would relate this to the need to control children at meal times. There was also a class difference in whether meals were eaten at table with the likelihood of the whole family eating at table being greatest in classes I and II. This is shown in Table 8.7.

Table 8.7 *Main meal eaten at table by men's occupational class – no. (%)*

	Sunday main meal	Weekday main meal	Weekday main meal and non-main meal	Breakfast
I/II	55 (92)	47 (78)	40 (67)	48 (80)
IIIN	24 (86)	20 (71)	17 (61)	17 (61)
IIIM	65 (83)	60 (77)	47 (60)	45 (58)
IV/V	16 (76)	14 (67)	12 (57)	14 (67)
No partner	5 (50)	4 (40)	5 (50)	4 (40)
Student	2 (67)	2 (67)	2 (67)	2 (67)

It seems to us from going into women's homes that this class difference can at least partly be explained by the space available for eating. In some homes, particularly those of families with little money, it was often impossible for the family to eat at table. Some kitchens were simply too small to fit a table into and there was no space for putting a dining table in the living room. Some families, although having a table in the kitchen, were too numerous to be able to sit at it comfortably together and this meant that meals had to be eaten in the sitting room. Often younger children ate at the table while the older children ate off their knees. The pressure of space was not the same in better off families where houses often boasted spacious kitchens as well as a dining room. One woman described the problems that lack of space created. Her partner ate his meal in front of the television while she and her two children ate at the tiny kitchen table.

That's a bit of a daft performance, 'cos he puts telly on and kids are straining their neck round door, you see, to watch television and I'm saying, 'You get on with your tea', 'Yeah but I'm just watching that' and I'm saying, 'Michael, will you switch the telly off,' 'No, I'm listening to news,' and you know it's a bit of a bind really.

The whole order and discipline of a mealtime could therefore be lost due to lack of space for all the family to eat at the table. It could also be lost through children wanting to copy their dads' behaviour. One woman recounted her lost battles to get her daughter to eat at table. She was asked where they normally ate.

In here on trays. He doesn't like eating at table and she won't if he doesn't so I don't bother. The kitchen isn't big enough either to eat in – I don't think. We have to pull the table out. I can't make her eat in the kitchen if we don't – she likes to watch telly and I don't mind. [Does she sit on the floor?] Yeah, she has a stool. We should really sit at table – when we get a bigger house we might do, you know. If I make her sit at table she'd just leave it whereas she eats it if she's sat in here with us.

And even when men were not present to set a bad example mealtimes were often more disorganised than women would have liked them to be. One woman who was a single parent said that she didn't like anyone to read at mealtimes.

I like it when we can all sit down together actually like, I think it's when they're at school and I get organised 'cos I like us all to sit together at teatime if we can. As I say it isn't always like that during the holidays. It doesn't seem to be so organised really. I mean I like us all to sit down together, you know.

In households where there was space to eat together at table mealtimes tended to be more organised and this usually (but not always) coincided with differences in occupational class. Eating a meal together, then, did not necessarily mean that everyone sat round the same table, nor did it always mean that everyone ate the same food. In some families women found themselves cooking two or three different meals at the same time. This happened if children had particular likes and dislikes which were then catered for by providing them with different meals. One woman described how she fed her family of four children and father-in-law as well as herself and her partner. She and one of the children preferred 'English' food while her partner and the other children would eat 'Chinese' or 'savoury' foods.

Sometimes I might do them one meal and us another meal, I don't like savouries so I might do half a savoury meal and half a plain meal and half'll have the savoury meal and half'll have the plain meal . . . It doesn't bother me doing that . . . I don't do my own chips because I can't be bothered. I find that one might want chips and one might not, so I just put my hand in [the freezer] and get a few chips out.

As she indicates, this sort of practice lends itself to reliance on convenience foods of one sort or another and seemed to be more common in working-class households.

Talking at meals

There were other differences in mealtimes between households which related to the importance attached to meals as a time for people to talk to each other. For example some families watched television or listened to the radio during meals and others didn't. Many women differentiated a Sunday meal from meals during the rest of the week by serving it at table and turning off the television. So even if meals were not eaten at table and people did not talk to each other because they were watching television for most of the time, on a Sunday a special effort was made to create a 'family' meal.

One of the women told us that the radio or television was always on during mealtimes 'except Sunday dinner, and then I switch them all off for some strange reason'. She went on,

I sound very domineering don't I? I've been brought up on a family meal every day. Now I aren't against Alan doing things his way but I believe that the children should experience a family meal, that's why I sometimes have a meal in the kitchen. [So if you have a family meal everything is turned off and you talk, do you?] Yes, for most of it, yes.

Most women felt that talking and exchanging news were important parts of mealtimes. Of the women 127 (63·5%) said that they thought it was important to talk at mealtimes while only 38 (19%) said it was not important. There was a significant class difference in the attitude to talking at mealtimes with 81% of women in classes I/II regarding it as important compared to 60% of women in class IIIN, 62% of women in class IIIM and 56% of women in classes IV and V. Conversely, while 33% of women in classes IV and V thought talking was positively not important and even detrimental to the business of eating, only 7% of women in classes I/II adopted this view.

It is interesting that talking at mealtimes was viewed by some women as an obstacle in the way of eating and by others as a means by which children might be encouraged to eat; this was linked to social class. For example, a woman from social class I said: 'I think it's [talking] a very important part of getting the children to eat well actually.'

In contrast to this a woman from class IIIM said:

... I've played pop with the kids because sometimes they're talking more often than they're eating. When I was young I wasn't allowed to speak at table, which I wasn't. It was sit down, eat your meal and then 'can I leave the table', when we were little. We could never speak unless we were spoken to. And I think now, I think well I'm not going to be so strict with my kids, but sometimes I will say to them, 'now shut up and get on with your tea', or lunch or whatever, you see.

Many of the women clearly felt mealtimes were important occasions for the family as a unit. One woman was asked: 'Do you think it's important to talk together at family mealtimes?' She replied:

Yeah. When the father's out at work all day, luckily with him being able to be at home all weekend they can build up a father–daughter relationship that's pretty strong and he does get on well with the children. I mean some fathers don't necessarily get on very well with their children just because they can't communicate but for the children's sake if they are not really included in the conversation at times like meals I sort of wonder what do they really feel, what do they really think ... Quite often at mealtimes it's a chance for Jon and I to talk about something ... I've discovered in a lot of ways that if we're all sat at the table at mealtimes Jon and I can talk and have a much more sensible conversation than we would at any other time.

In some families there seem to be the remnants of the Victorian dictum that children 'should be seen and not heard', although this was true in only a small proportion, mainly in social classes IIIM, IV and V. There was also a different standard applied to adults and children in these families. One woman said:

I don't even like people talking. If I'm out in company that's fair enough but I don't like kiddies talking when they're eating. I just like to eat the meal – I don't mean that I don't like people to say something but mine will start to tell you something that's happened at school and it's right drawn out. Joanna will be sat there with her knife and fork poised for about ten minutes while she's telling you something and that aggravates me, so personally I like to eat the meal in silence.

Radio and television

Having the television or radio on during meals reduces conversation and so we might expect to find that I/II families were less likely to eat their meals in the company of the television than others. In fact, amongst the sample as a whole the majority of families had the television on during at least some meals and the same was true of the radio. In only about a third of the families were meals never accompanied by television watching or radio listening and if the radio was on it was more likely to be at breakfast than any other meal.

What is interesting is that if the meal was eaten at table and was regarded as a family meal it was less likely to be accompanied by the radio or television. Thus several women told us that they only ate with the television on if they were eating in the sitting room. In other families, meals were only eaten in front of the television if there was something that someone particularly wanted to see. But in many families children's programmes were on during mealtimes and this could cause problems, particularly if they coincided with a main meal. 'Unfortunately yes . . . the television usually. 'Cos usually by the time we're eating it's their cartoons and bits and pieces that they like which I will switch off but some people prefer them to watch them.' And in other families women insisted on the television being switched off because it distracted children from eating. 'This is why we've started eating in there 'cos I won't allow her to watch television now. It sounds a bit strict but I can't stand them leaving the meal and "Oh it's cold" because she's been trying to watch that.' There was considerable difference between what happened at the main, proper meal and other meals. Indeed it sometimes seemed that part of a proper meal was that it should be a time when television and radio were off. Many families had the television on during the weekday meals but not for the proper meal par excellence on a Sunday.

There are, as we suggested above, class differences in television watching at mealtimes. This is true for both women's and men's occupational class. Nearly half the families in occupational classes I/II *never* had the television on during mealtimes compared with less than a third of families in other occupational classes. Interestingly, class I/II families are much more likely to have the radio on at breakfast than other families although they are less frequent radio listeners at other mealtimes.

From this evidence there does seem to emerge a class variation in mealtimes which suggests that mealtimes – at least main mealtimes –might be more formal and organised in households from the higher occupational classes than in others. There seems, in every class, to be great importance attached to the family meal on a Sunday, but on weekdays the form that the main meal of the day takes is more variable and depends on the place occupied by the family (particularly the man at this stage in the life cycle) in the occupational hierarchy.

'Table manners'

Talking and having a family meal were also seen as important for encouraging children to have good table manners; it was an important part of the socialisation process. One of the women said:

I think [talking] is important for the children's table manners as well . . . I think if children eat separately from their parents or the father eats differently, you often find that fathers eat later at night, don't you, from everybody else, I think it's a family thing and I don't think that you can check your children and see that their table manners . . . if you're not there to supervise it.

Practically all the women thought that table manners were important (170 – 85%). The most commonly mentioned were encouraging the children to say please and thank you (174 – 87%), encouraging them to use utensils correctly (168 – 84%), encouraging them not to bring books and toys to table (143 – 71·5%), encouraging them not to make a noise at table (137 – 68·5%) and encouraging them to ask permission to leave the table (108 – 54%). Only one of the women said that table manners were not important. But sometimes it was difficult to teach children manners, for instance one woman said: 'We don't sit at table so how can she have table manners?' And this clearly related to occupational class. It is difficult, if not impossible, to teach a child table manners if meals are not usually eaten at table.

Again, when discussing manners, the distinction between weekdays and Sunday eating emerged; this distinction operated throughout the occupational structure. One woman said:

> I think perhaps if I had put a cloth on the table and we were having a Sunday lunch – I think I'd make a distinction between the ordinary meals when we sit at the table and just mats and a family atmosphere and a meal where perhaps I'd decided that we were going to have a cloth and nice utensils and a sit down meal and then I think I would expect the sort of manners that I might expect if I took him out. Perhaps a bit later on, at the moment I don't expect anything really of a child under two.

Table manners were generally seen as being important to a family meal where everyone is eating together and, supposedly, enjoying their food. This is often difficult when meals are eaten with young children and perhaps explains some adults' prefer-ence for eating later in the evening after their children have gone to bed, at least until they have learnt to eat properly. One woman described the drawbacks of eating with young children.

> . . . obviously when you're eating as a family you want to eat your meal and be able to enjoy it, if a child's picking up food with their fingers and putting it in their mouth and then it isn't particularly pleasant to be sat opposite them watching them mangle all their food.

Perhaps this also partly explains some men's preference to eat their meals in the company of the television rather than their children! Children needed to be taught to eat properly – by women – so that their eating behaviour was socially acceptable. The acquisition of table manners was seen as an important part of this process by most of the women although lack of a table to eat at, more common in working-class families, could make the process of socialisation into this mode of behaviour seem redundant.

There are clearly, then, class-specific modes of behaviour and ways of organising mealtimes with more middle-class families tending to have formal family meals than working-class fami-lies. So although proper meals and Sunday 'dinners' are an almost universal feature of family life, or are felt ideally to be part of it, practices within families depend to a large extent on their place in the occupational hierarchy. Children and adults from different class backgrounds therefore experience family eating differently and learn different modes of behaviour. And the constraints women experience in their attempts to feed their families properly also vary with social class. This results not only in a different organisation and experience of meals but also in different foods going to make up those meals. Class variation in food consumption will therefore be the starting point of the next chapter.

9

Class, food consumption and hospitality

Husband: I have a thing about chips. I can't rationalise it. I always feel that chips are associated with the lower classes. I've got this thing about – I hate the smell of chips, the cooking smell associated with it . . . I've always thought – do I dare say it? – it smells like a council house when you come in and it stinks of chips – that's awful isn't it? Some of our best friends live in council houses – never mind. I just associate it with cheap and nasty to be honest with you . . . I associate chips with slap happy cooking, you know, like I say, cheap and nasty.

[When you were still working and married to your first husband, did you cook different things from what you cook now?] Yes, completely different because he was a very different eater. He ate a lot of chips and fried things. I used to cook loads and loads of fried things, and loads of horrible fatty, starchy things, white bread, he was completely different . . . just had an ordinary sort of a job as a bus driver, you know, then I met Simon, he was at university and he came from a well-to-do family with money . . . When I first started living with Simon, we both decided not to fry so many things and I recognise food values more . . . he ate better than me so when we started living together I just went onto what he liked.

Food, and the way it is presented, conveys messages about the social status of those participating in meals. These messages can be read and understood by all of us (provided we are members of the same culture) even though we may not be consciously aware that this is what is happening. The quotes above for instance seem to tell us that working-class diets are likely to include large amounts of chips and other fried food whereas middle-class diets will not rely so much on fried foods but will be 'better' in nutritional terms. If this is so, it means that the food we eat conveys messages which are part of our taken-for-granted social existence; we never stop to think about them, but we all know what they mean. But how far are differences of class and status actually reflected in the foods that we eat? How do social relations and divisions affect our diets? Are our preconceptions based on real differences or are they prejudices and stereotypes that people from different social backgrounds hold about each other? This is what we wish to explore in this chapter and to do so we shall look at two specific areas of family eating. Firstly, we shall explore the actual frequency with which certain foods are eaten by people in different social classes, and then we shall look at class variations in the role played by food when offering hospitality to visiting family and friends.

Diet

Throughout the class structure women regarded the proper meal as the basis of proper, family eating. We would therefore expect, if families' eating patterns conformed to women's aspirations, that the consumption of meat and fish, potatoes and cooked vegetables would be fairly uniform. As we can see from Table 9.1 this is by and large the case. However, high status meat is eaten most frequently by women, men and children in occupational class IIIM and is eaten less frequently by adults in occupational classes I/II and IV/V than by those in the intermediate classes. High status meat, while regarded as being of good quality and therefore socially desirable, was expensive and families on low incomes were not able to afford it very often. For most families it constituted the joint for Sunday lunch twice during the diary fortnight and one or two other meals might be steak or chops or chicken. Those on low incomes, even if they wanted to eat this sort of meat more often, and from what the women told us it seemed that they did, were constrained by its high cost and did not buy it as often as other families who had more money coming into the household. This undoubtedly explained its lower consumption in class IV/V families. However, adults in households in occupational classes I/II also ate high status meat less often and this cannot usually be explained by lack of money. We would argue that here the presence of

Table 9.1   *Average number of times specific foods eaten during diary fortnight, by occupational class (defined according to the women's current or last full-time occupation; figures in brackets represent class patterns of consumption defined by men's occupation)*

	Women	Men	Children
High status meat			
I/II	4·2 (4·4)	4·4 (4·4)	3·1 (3·1)
IIIN	4·5 (4·4)	4·9 (4·9)	3·1 (3·0)
IIIM	4·7 (4·7)	5·5 (5·1)	3·2 (3·2)
IV/V	4·4 (4·3)	4·7 (4·3)	2·8 (3·0)
Medium status meat			
I/II	6·6 (6·0)	7·7 (6·7)	5·7 (5·6)
IIIN	7·0 (6·9)	9·4 (9·3)	5·2 (4·8)
IIIM	6·4 (7·4)	10·4 (9·3)	5·5 (5·3)
IV/V	5·8 (6·0)	6·2 (10·5)	4·4 (5·3)
Whole fish			
I/II	1·2 (1·8)	1·6 (1·6)	0·7 (1·1)
IIIN	1·8 (2·0)	1·9 (2·7)	0·9 (1·0)
IIIM	1·9 (1·7)	2·6 (1·8)	1·2 (0·9)
IV/V	1·9 (0·9)	1·8 (1·4)	0·7 (0·6)
Potatoes			
I/II	6·9 (6·7)	6·9 (6·2)	6·4 (6·2)
IIIN	6·4 (6·2)	6·5 (6·6)	6·2 (6·6)
IIIM	6·1 (6·3)	6·6 (6·8)	6·2 (6·8)
IV/V	6·0 (6·1)	6·0 (5·9)	5·9 (5·9)
All cooked vegetables			
I/II	10·3 (9·9)	10·4 (8·9)	8·3 (8·0)
IIIN	11·0 (10·6)	11·0 (11·6)	8·9 (8·5)
IIIM	10·1 (11·1)	11·5 (11·7)	8·4 (9·1)
IV/V	11·4 (11·4)	11·1 (10·9)	8·0 (8·5)

alternative food ideologies, which had led four of the families to become vegetarian, are important, together with the greater significance of nutritional factors in determining the food that these families ate. One woman from this occupational class explained to us the changes she had made in her own and her family's diet:

We always used to have the evening meal based on meat in some way, we'd eat meat every day. We used to eat a lot of eggs for breakfast, white bread, sugary puddings. What I suppose it was was the food of your childhood, the food of your childhood strained through the French cookery books – kind of up-market, that sort of thing – with curries and a certain amount of Italian influence on it.

A typical meal for them now would be: 'Baked potato with grated cheese and cottage cheese and we ate carrot, parsnip and broccoli and we ate a pear each for pudding.' She described their diet as being 'within the accepted mores of a whole food vegetarian diet . . . though probably deficient in the lentils and pulses department'. It seemed to us from talking to the women that those in occupational class I/II families did not attach quite so much importance to meat as did women from more working-class backgrounds. Also, families in occupational class I/II ate cooked vegetables less often than others, indicating that other types of meal might be acceptable as alternatives to the proper meal. And meals might often be egg or cheese based or include beans or other pulses without this being felt as a social deprivation. Also, spaghetti and other pasta and rice based meals were more frequent and took the place of the traditional meat and two veg., whereas in more working-class households the *structure* of the proper meal was maintained even though the constituent elements might not be 'proper'. Thus, beans, sausages and chips might be a substitute in a working-class household on a low income whereas a cheese omelette, salad and wholemeal bread might take its place in a household that was more middle-class; or if sausages were eaten they would be more likely to be accompanied by fresh vegetables and boiled potatoes. Both could be regarded as a response to the expense of good quality meat but they have different social, and nutritional, implications. One middle-class woman was reduced to feeding her son on egg and chips because it was the only meal that he would eat. She told us how she felt:

When he started on solid food he just had what we had mashed and he enjoyed it, he used to eat curry and all sorts as a baby. Then at some point along the line . . . he just suddenly decided he wasn't going to eat anything of that sort again and for a year or more it was just egg and chips. I was bitterly ashamed to keep serving up – particularly if people came, like the insurance man used to come and there would be this awful child sitting at the table eating egg and chips and I'd think he thought, 'What a dreadful woman, how lazy', which is what I would have thought had I not known.

She was ashamed to be seen feeding him in this way because the meal was not a 'proper' meal, she was not feeding him 'properly'. But perhaps there is also in this guilt the feeling that it is the 'lower classes' who eat in this way and the provision of this food is somehow also inappropriate for that reason.

In Table 9.2 the foods that are eaten as an alternative to the proper meal are shown and there clearly are class differences in the frequency with which they are eaten. Cheese, pulses and nuts, and pasta and rice are eaten much more often in households in occupational classes I/II then in the other classes, while chips and tinned baked beans, etc., are eaten much less frequently in these households. Eggs and low status meat/fish do not show any clear class pattern except that men in occupational classes I/II eat less low status meat or fish than men in other classes.

Chips are eaten least often by women, men and children in occupational classes I/II, but children's and women's consumption increases and is highest in occupational classes IV/V, while men's is highest in occupational class IIIM. This ties in with comments made by women whose partners were working-class. One, who had recently separated from her partner, told us that he had insisted on fry-ups: 'He was a fry-up, always fried foods, all the time, greasy foods, always the same thing . . . ' Many women found it difficult to feed their families on less fatty food because of their partners' preference for chips and other fried foods. So men's preferences again seem to be important. Through their influence on what other members of their families eat, their preferences also shape class patterns of eating.

The class distribution of these foods supports the view that the alternatives to the proper meal are different in the different classes even though it forms the basis of the majority of families' diets throughout the class structure.

Milk, fresh fruit and fresh vegetables were foods which, along with meat, were regarded by many women on low incomes as too expensive for them to buy regularly. They were also highly regarded as being 'good for you' and, especially, as being important for children. Table 9.3 shows the differences in frequency of consumption of these foods, and all of them were eaten much more often by families in occupational classes I/II

Table 9.2 *Average number of times specific foods eaten during diary fortnight by occupational class. ('Baked beans, etc.' includes such things as Noodle Doodles, tinned spaghetti, tinned ravioli, etc.)*

	Women	Men	Children
Foods eaten most often by families in occupational classes I/II			
Cheese			
I/II	7·1 (7·4)	7·1 (7·6)	5·6 (4·9)
IIIN	5·3 (6·8)	5·7 (5·8)	3·6 (4·1)
IIIM	4·9 (4·3)	4·9 (4·9)	2·9 (3·1)
IV/V	4·1 (3·9)	4·4 (3·6)	1·3 (2·4)
Pulses and nuts			
I/II	1·3 (0·9)	0·7 (0·6)	0·7 (0·4)
IIIN	0·0 (0·1)	0·0 (0·1)	0·0 (0·1)
IIIM	0·0 (0·1)	0·1 (0·1)	0·0 (0·0)
IV/V	0·1 (0·0)	0·2 (0·0)	0·0 (0·0)
Pasta/rice			
I/II	2·0 (1·4)	1·9 (1·8)	1·5 (1·4)
IIIN	0·5 (0·7)	0·9 (1·2)	0·5 (0·7)
IIIM	0·5 (0·3)	1·1 (0·9)	0·5 (0·3)
IV/V	0·4 (0·6)	1·3 (0·9)	0·4 (0·6)
Foods eaten least often by families in occupational classes I/II			
Chips			
I/II	2·9 (3·4)	1·7 (1·4)	2·9 (2·8)
IIIN	4·7 (4·2)	5·4 (5·6)	4·2 (3·8)
IIIM	5·3 (4·7)	6·2 (5·7)	4·3 (4·5)
IV/V	5·7 (5·3)	5·7 (5·5)	5·4 (4·6)
Tinned baked beans, etc.			
I/II	1·5 (1·6)	1·7 (1·4)	2·3 (2·6)
IIIN	2·0 (1·6)	2·2 (1·7)	3·0 (2·4)
IIIM	2·0 (2·0)	2·2 (2·1)	3·2 (3·1)
IV/V	2·6 (2·8)	1·8 (3·4)	3·6 (3·8)
Food showing no clear class pattern			
Eggs			
I/II	4·2 (4·0)	5·1 (4·4)	3·5 (2·7)
IIIN	4·4 (5·5)	5·2 (5·9)	3·2 (3·9)
IIIM	4·8 (4·3)	5·1 (5·2)	4·0 (3·8)
IV/V	3·8 (4·6)	4·4 (4·7)	3·2 (3·9)
Low status meat/fish			
I/II	4·5 (4·4)	5·2 (4·8)	5·2 (4·6)
IIIN	5·4 (6·5)	7·2 (8·4)	5·4 (7·1)
IIIM	4·6 (5·1)	7·1 (7·3)	5·0 (5·6)
IV/V	5·2 (4·0)	7·6 (6·4)	6·1 (3·8)

Table 9.3 *Average number of times specific foods eaten during diary fortnight by occupational class. Fresh fruit, raw vegetables and milk*

	Women	Men	Children
Fresh fruit			
I/II	10·0 (9·1)	7·9 (7·0)	11·8 (11·1)
IIIN	5·6 (4·5)	4·6 (5·1)	6·6 (5·8)
IIIM	4·1 (4·3)	4·8 (3·9)	5·9 (5·5)
IV/V	3·6 (4·3)	2·0 (4·8)	3·5 (5·4)
Raw vegetables			
I/II	6·4 (6·7)	7·1 (6·6)	3·8 (3·3)
IIIN	4·7 (5·9)	4·9 (7·5)	1·9 (3·0)
IIIM	5·9 (4·4)	5·6 (4·2)	2·7 (1·9)
IV/V	2·7 (3·2)	3·0 (3·0)	0·9 (1·4)
Milk			
I/II	9·2 (9·1)	8·9 (9·0)	22·6 (24·1)
IIIN	5·6 (4·8)	5·9 (6·1)	22·4 (19·6)
IIIM	4·1 (4·8)	4·9 (4·7)	20·5 (21·4)
IV/V	3·6 (4·1)	4·3 (4·3)	17·2 (19·3)

than other families. Although income is probably important here, we also feel that the dominance of the proper meal as the major structuring element of the diet is significant. Fresh fruit and uncooked vegetables are not constituent parts of the proper meal, nor of breakfast or the non-main meal, although a 'traditional' Sunday tea may include a salad. In families where the proper meal is not considered to be vital, at least as it is understood by most women as meat or fish, potatoes and *cooked* vegetables, salad may be an acceptable substitute for cooked vegetables and fresh fruit may be an acceptable substitute for pudding. This seemed a more common practice in households in occupational classes I/II than others. This can also be related to the apparently greater significance of nutritional considerations in these families and the influence of non-British traditions of eating which seem to have had more impact in some sectors of occupational classes I/II than in the other occupational classes.

Breakfast and the non-main meal, unlike the main meal, are bread and cereal-based meals and although the frequency of bread consumption does not show any class variation, the type of bread that is eaten does: 48% of occupational class I/II families ate wholemeal bread compared with 13% of those in class IIIN, 10% of those in IIIM and 6% in classes IV and V. In contrast, 7% of class I/II families ate white bread compared with 37% in class IIIN, 41% in class IIIM and 67% in classes IV and V. (This is according to women's occupational class.) We would again relate this to the impact of nutritional thinking and income; wholemeal bread is not as cheap as Mother's Pride sliced white! In Table 9.4 bread and breakfast cereal consumption is shown and it can be seen that breakfast cereal is eaten more frequently by women and men in occupational classes I/II than any other class, although children's consumption does not show the same pattern.

Table 9.4 *Average number of times specific foods eaten during diary fortnight by occupational class. Bread and breakfast cereal*

	Women	Men	Children
Bread			
I/II	18·5 (19·6)	20·0 (20·0)	20·3 (19·4)
IIIN	20·0 (21·0)	22·3 (23·2)	17·1 (17·2)
IIIM	17·0 (18·1)	22·0 (21·3)	14·3 (17·0)
IV/V	17·1 (16·8)	20·4 (21·2)	16·6 (14·2)
Breakfast cereal			
I/II	8·2 (7·6)	7·9 (8·3)	10·7 (11·9)
IIIN	4·7 (4·2)	5·2 (4·9)	10·5 (10·9)
IIIM	3·6 (4·1)	4·1 (4·0)	10·7 (9·4)
IV/V	3·5 (3·9)	2·4 (2·9)	9·4 (10·9)

Foods that are eaten for pleasure and are not considered to be an essential part of a healthy diet are generally sweet foods and their consumption is shown in Table 9.5. Biscuits and cake do not show very clear class patterns, except that adults in occupational classes IV/V eat biscuits less often than other adults, but the consumption of puddings and sweets does. Puddings are eaten most often by women, men and children in occupational classes I/II and least often in occupational classes IV/V. Women's and men's sweet consumption does not show a clear pattern but children's sweet consumption is greatest in occupational classes IIIN and IIIM and the class differences are clearest if women's occupational class is taken as the measure.

Table 9.5 *Average number of times specific foods eaten during diary fortnight by occupational class. Cake, puddings, biscuits and sweets*

	Women	Men	Children
Cake			
I/II	7·4 (6·9)	7·3 (6·5)	6·1 (5·7)
IIIN	7·0 (5·7)	7·5 (5·2)	5·1 (3·9)
IIIM	5·3 (6·7)	7·5 (8·0)	3·9 (4·7)
IV/V	5·1 (6·3)	5·3 (6·9)	3·4 (4·5)
Puddings			
I/II	9·1 (8·9)	7·7 (8·1)	11·1 (12·3)
IIIN	7·2 (8·7)	7·0 (8·9)	9·8 (10·5)
IIIM	5·7 (6·1)	6·9 (5·7)	8·3 (8·2)
IV/V	5·3 (5·8)	6·1 (5·8)	6·5 (6·8)
Biscuits			
I/II	9·7 (10·1)	7·2 (6·8)	11·8 (13·8)
IIIN	8·9 (7·0)	7·0 (7·2)	12·4 (9·7)
IIIM	5·7 (7·6)	5·0 (5·9)	11·0 (10·8)
IV/V	3·4 (6·3)	3·0 (5·1)	5·9 (9·9)
Sweets			
I/II	3·6 (4·9)	2·3 (3·3)	6·9 (7·8)
IIIN	3·8 (2·4)	2·9 (2·3)	8·9 (7·9)
IIIM	3·4 (3·1)	2·0 (2·1)	8·8 (8·8)
IV/V	2·1 (3·0)	1·9 (1·9)	6·8 (7·7)

There seems to be more of a class difference in the *reported* frequency of giving sweets to children. In occupational classes I/II 26% of women gave their children sweets on a daily basis compared with 50% of women in class IIIN, 55% of women in class IIIM and 50% of women in classes IV and V. In addition, the only women who reported that they never gave their children sweets were in occupational classes I/II. Qualitative accounts also suggest that these children are more likely to receive only one or two sweets at a time whereas children in other social classes may receive a whole packet to eat at once. A woman in social class I, for instance, said:

Of course, people often come to the house and present your children with sweets and it is the custom in this house, we have a sweet cupboard, and they are always allowed to take one or two out of the top of the packet of the gift and then one of them brings the packet to me and I put it in the cupboard. They can generally have something if they ask for it.

This woman is clearly in control of what her children eat between meals. A woman in occupational class IIIN said that her children had 'a drink of juice and a packet of Rolos or Smarties or something in the morning', and 'a packet of sweets each in the afternoon'. Sweet consumption appears to be most frequent amongst the children of women in occupational class IIIM. One woman, who was married to a manual worker, said: 'It's pretty natural for them to have sweets, it's the normal thing, it's not a treat 'cos they get them every day.'

This sort of attitude was typical in all classes apart from I and II where sweet consumption was lowest. It was also lower in classes IV and V and women's accounts suggest that this is the result of low income; children are given sweets in these households whenever they can be afforded. In classes I/II the reasons for lower sweet consumption are different. There seems to be more effective control over between-meal eating by the mother and a different attitude towards treating children. It seems that children in other social classes are treated with sweets and indulged as far as the means of the family will allow and that this does not occur to nearly such an extent in class I/II.

Drinks

Drinks such as tea and coffee and soft drinks show little variation with occupational class, at least as far as adults' consumption is concerned. This is shown in Table 9.6. Children's consumption of tea and coffee, however, is lowest in occupational classes I/II and highest in occupational classes IV/V. This is a reflection of the practice, which was fairly common in working-class households, of giving children very milky tea or coffee to drink and of giving it to them in their bottles. This did not happen so often in middle-class households, where children were much more likely to be given milk. This also ties in with the higher milk consumption among children in occupational classes I/II which we noted earlier.

Adults' alcohol consumption, however, shows quite a marked variation with occupational class, with the highest rates of consumption to be found in occupational classes I/II and the

Table 9.6 *Average number of times specific foods eaten during diary fortnight by occupational class. Soft drinks, tea, coffee and alcohol*

	Women	Men	Children
Soft drinks			
I/II	2·0 (2·7)	1·3 (1·8)	24·2 (26·1)
IIIN	3·2 (3·1)	2·2 (2·3)	23·7 (27·6)
IIIM	2·2 (3·0)	2·2 (1·7)	24·6 (19·8)
IV/V	2·6 (1·4)	3·2 (3·2)	13·6 (20·1)
Tea/coffee			
I/II	54·6 (58·2)	51·0 (54·8)	5·9 (7·2)
IIIN	57·9 (55·4)	56·2 (51·6)	14·9 (9·4)
IIIM	61·3 (57·1)	54·3 (53·0)	16·2 (16·6)
IV/V	59·8 (59·1)	45·7 (47·1)	21·0 (19·7)
Alcohol			
I/II	3·9 (3·8)	5·4 (5·8)	0·2 (0·2)
IIIN	2·7 (3·2)	4·3 (5·3)	0·2 (0·3)
IIIM	1·2 (2·5)	3·1 (3·6)	0·1 (0·1)
IV/V	2·4 (1·0)	2·6 (1·5)	0·3 (0·0)

lowest in IV/V. Children hardly drink it at all. Patterns of drinking at home and drinking in the pub are closely related to class, with middle-class men and women being most likely to drink at home and least likely to drink at the pub. Working-class women seemed to drink alcohol very infrequently, perhaps because drinking at home was not a common occurrence and going to the pub was difficult for women who had young children to look after; a constraint that their partners did not seem to suffer from! Indeed, it seemed to be an accepted part of male, working-class culture to go for a few pints after work was over or, more usually, after the evening meal. One woman told us that her partner felt under pressure to indulge in this sort of drinking even though he was not very keen on beer. After a 2 till 10 shift his workmates 'badgered' him to have a drink with them. She told us: 'I always say to him you should only have a half but it's not very manly to only have a half, he's got to have the big one. Got to keep up with everybody else.' This drinking at the pub with your mates seems to be part of working-class masculinity, whereas in middle-class, particularly professional, homes men and women might have a drink together during the evening, perhaps on returning home from work to revive flagging spirits. However, even among occupational class I/II families, this was not a very widespread practice. It was more usual to have a bottle of wine at the weekend, either with a meal on Saturday evening after the children had gone to bed or with the Sunday roast. One woman said: 'We have several racks of wine in the house but we only open it when we have people in. However we often reel in from work and pour ourselves a gin.' And it almost goes without saying, such are the messages that drinking habits convey, that this was a middle-class professional household.

Table 9.7 *Occasions alcohol drunk at home by men's occupational class (n = 197) – no. (%) (Percentages do not always total 100)*

	I/II		IIIN		IIIM		IV/V		Single Parent		Total	
Christmas and special occasions	4	(7)	3	(11)	24	(31)	9	(43)	2	(20)	42	(21)
Christmas, special occasions and when having company	6	(10)	5	(18)	7	(9)	4	(19)	2	(20)	24	(12)
At other times but not frequently	24	(40)	14	(50)	22	(28)	4	(19)	1	(10)	65	(33)
Once a week or more	20	(33)	5	(18)	11	(14)	2	(10)	–		38	(19)
Never drink at home	1	(2)	–		3	(4)	1	(5)	2	(20)	7	(3)
Other/not given	5	(8)	1	(4)	11	(14)	1	(5)	3	(30)	21	(11)
Total	60	(100)	28	(100)	78	(100)	21	(100)	10	(100)	197	(100)

The figures for alcohol consumption at home can be seen in Table 9.7. The reason we are using men's occupational class to analyse alcohol consumption is that it seems to be something that was much more associated with men than women, even to the extent that men were much more likely than women to buy alcoholic drinks, to suggest when they were drunk and to pour them out. Alcohol provision was largely a man's domain in the same way that food provision was woman's domain, although, as with shopping for food, men and women were more likely to share buying of alcohol in occupational classes I/II. Drinking at the pub was similarly more of a masculine than feminine pursuit. Substantial numbers of men in all occupational classes went out to the pub without their partners whereas this was extremely uncommon amongst the women and almost totally confined to those living as single parents. In all occupational classes about half of the men and women tended to go to the pub together and in all the classes except I/II the proportion of men going to the pub without their partners was only slightly lower. The proportion of men in occupational classes I/II who go alone to the pub is much lower than in the other classes. This is shown in Table 9.8.

Table 9.8 *Pub drinking by men's occupational class – no. (%)* *(Percentages do not always total 100)*

	I/II	IIIN	IIIM	IV/V	Single parent	Total
Both go to pub	32 (53)	16 (57)	38 (49)	10 (48)	–	96 (49)
Men go alone	17 (28)	12 (43)	33 (42)	9 (43)	–	71 (36)
Women go alone	–	–	1 (1)	–	7 (70)	8 (4)
Neither go to pub	9 (15)	–	5 (6)	1 (5)	–	15 (8)
No information	2 (3)	–	1 (1)	1 (5)	3 (30)	7 (3)
Total	60 (100)	28 (100)	78 (100)	21 (100)	10 (100)	197 (100)

It seems then that occupational class has a significant effect on drinking habits and that it also influences gender divisions. Men and women in occupational classes I/II seem to be more likely to drink together at home or go out to the pub together, whereas in other social classes men's and women's spheres seem to be much more clearly demarcated from each other. Indeed, women's attitudes to men's drinking seemed to depend to a large extent on their class. In the working-class it was much more accepted that men should go out on their own, whereas middle-class women expected, and usually seemed to get, equal participation in outings to the pub and drinking in general. A middle-class woman, for instance, told us that her partner used to go to the pub quite often with friends but: 'I started to object rather violently because I didn't have anybody to go out with, they were his friends . . . I wouldn't have objected if I had been going out by myself but on the whole it was people looking for him . . . Now friends tend to come round more.' Whereas a working-class woman said:

We seem to go in spurts. We go out quite a lot and then don't go out for a couple of weeks. Phil goes out every Friday night though. I think it's important to him 'cos I think once you start stopping a man going out you've had it really, haven't you? I think you have because I've heard it so many times from one or two of my friends, 'Oh I'm not letting my husband out', and the following year they've been divorced, you know. I always think that what you don't know you don't worry about do you?

There seemed to be an expectation of a more egalitarian partnership, at least in terms of drinking and going out together, in occupational class I/II families than in others and it is interesting to see whether this different form of gender division is reflected in food consumption. As we saw earlier, certain foods are eaten more often by men than women and others are eaten more often by women than men. Do these differences vary with occupational class or are they constant throughout the class structure? In other words, does occupational class affect the form taken by gender divisions?

Gender divisions and class

In order to explore this issue we will look at the consumption of meat, alcohol and cake, as these were identified as being 'status' foods which show different rates of consumption according to gender. To show the extent of gender differences in frequency of consumption we have taken women's consumption to be 100 in every social class. This is shown in Table 9.9

Gender differences in meat consumption appear to be least marked in occupational classes I/II although men consume meat more frequently than women in every occupational class. The only exception to this is in classes I/II and IV/V according to men's occupational class where gender differences in frequency of consumption of high status meat disappear. Cake consumption

Table 9.9 *Gender differences in average frequency of consumption of meat, cake and alcohol by women's occupational class. (Figures for men's occupational class in brackets)*

	Women	Men	
High status meat			
I/II	100	105	(100)
IIIN	100	109	(111)
IIIM	100	117	(108)
IV/V	100	107	(100)
Medium status meat			
I/II	100	116	(101)
IIIN	100	134	(135)
IIIM	100	162	(145)
IV/V	100	107	(175)
Low status meat			
I/II	100	115	(109)
IIIN	100	133	(129)
IIIM	100	154	(143)
IV/V	100	146	(160)
Cake			
I/II	100	99	(94)
IIIN	100	107	(91)
IIIM	100	141	(119)
I/V	100	104	(109)
Alcohol			
I/II	100	138	(153)
IIIN	100	159	(165)
IIIM	100	258	(144)
IV/V	100	108	(150)

only shows a clear gender linkage in occupational classes IIIM, IV and V and we think that this difference is likely to be explained by the practice of putting cake in men's pack-ups, something which did not appear to happen, or happened to a lesser extent, in occupational classes I/II and IIIN. Alcohol consumption, despite the apparently more egalitarian drinking practices in occupational classes I/II shows large differences according to gender, with men in all occupational classes drinking significantly more frequently than women. So it seems that some gender divisions, as they are represented in food eaten and drink consumed, persist across the class structure while others are more marked in certain classes or are even specific to certain classes. Differences in adults' and children's food consumption also exist within each class and they show much less variation than gender differences. For instance, children in all occupational classes drink milk and eat breakfast cereal more often than adults and eat high status meat and drink alcohol less often.

The food and drink that people consume, therefore, is affected and to some extent determined by their position in the occupational hierarchy. But it is also influenced by their gender and their age. The opinions expressed at the beginning of the chapter on diets which are specifically working-class or middle-class are therefore not simply prejudice. Our analysis of families' actual food consumption shows that they are quite close to the way people in different classes actually eat. Vegetarians are more likely to come from the professional sector of occupational classes I/II, for instance, while men loving a big fry up are likely to be found among the manual working-class. Social divisions of class, as well as gender and age, shape the food people eat and the way that they eat it.

Hospitality

They also affect the way food is used as a sign of hospitality and, even, with whom meals are likely to be shared. Thus it is not only the way daily eating is organised that is affected by class, patterns of entertaining are also class-specific. For instance, a dinner party in the evening, with a three course meal and wine to which friends are invited and from which children are excluded, is much more likely to be given by a couple in occupational classes I/II, while sharing Sunday 'dinner' and 'tea' with parents and brothers and sisters, with children present, is much more likely to happen in a working-class than middle-class family. This difference can partly be linked to the fact that working-class men and women, at least in our sample, were much more likely to live close to their parents than men and women in occupational classes I/II. In the latter case, people had usually moved away from their parents either when they began higher education or with their jobs.

However, before we explore the sharing of meals with family and friends we think it is important to look at the way the offering of food and drink is used as a means of welcoming even the casual and unexpected visitor. And, conversely, if a cup of tea or coffee is not provided the visit is not likely to be a long one. Again, food is a means of conveying a message, in this case the message is about how welcome or unwelcome a visitor is, and it is a message which we can all read and understand.

Most of the families we talked to did not often go in for elaborate entertaining or frequent sharing of food with their friends. However, one of the women who did, spoke about the significance of food to social relations and we feel that she points to some important aspects of the place food occupies, usually unconsciously, in our social lives.

It's an excuse for a social gathering. I mean the meal to me is a focus ... On Midsummer's night ... we went out to this friend who lives in the country ... the function of food on that occasion was an important one because we started at half past nine and we finished when dawn broke and so the food was a sort of ... the food was a way in which we could be together.

She also felt that the provision of food could deflect a potentially difficult situation:

Well, at the weekend we had a good friend who's gone to America who was back here for just the weekend and we had a kind of breakfast party ... I sensed that the re-meeting of him ... might be problematic ... when this friend came from America ... I was anxious that there would be difficulties and therefore we established this rather elaborate breakfast, Sunday breakfast, because we could engage ourselves in the preparation and eating of that meal and wouldn't have to engage ourselves with a discussion of the problems ...

Her comments illustrate the importance of food to social relations in two very different circumstances, the first a celebratory meal with friends and the second a reunion with a friend who was staying with her after a long absence. In both cases food performed an important function which she clearly articulated. Most of the women we spoke to, however, did not analyse their use of food in this way; nonetheless their provision of it for visitors in their own homes performed similar functions and followed certain clear patterns depending on their relationship with and feelings towards their visitor/s. We will first explore the offering of food and drink to casual visitors and then go on to look at the provision of meals, such as Sunday dinner and tea, to family and friends and the laying on of dinner parties for friends and, very rarely, business friends.

About two-thirds of the way through the first interview we asked the women whether they offered food or drink to people dropping in. Their response was very interesting because it sometimes reminded them that they had not made us welcome in this way, and they broke off at this point to put the kettle on. Few women did not offer tea or coffee (or orange squash on hot summer days) to us. Those that did not were generally those who did not want the interview to last any longer than necessary and did not regard it as an at least potentially friendly exchange. Most women, however, offered us tea or coffee and often bisucits and home made cakes. Sometimes the best tea pot emerged to grace the occasion and trays were brought into the sitting room piled high with home made cakes. This provision, as well as being a sign of hospitality, was also a display of the fact that women were performing their role as provider of food and maintainer of high standards within the home. The best tea pot and home made cakes were an outward display of the status of the family, a form of conspicuous consumption.

Most of the women took it for granted that food or drink was offered to friends dropping in, indeed only two of them would not offer something to a visitor. Often what was offered depended on the time of day: 'Oh, yes, depending on what time of day it is, they usually have a drink, a cup of tea or a cup of coffee and a piece of cake or something.' Coffee was appropriate in the morning, tea in the afternoon and by the time evening came, an alcoholic drink could be offered.

Say a friend comes down on an evening, I mean you have to offer them a drink. Sometimes Gordon will ask them if they want a drink and sometimes people will say they would rather have a cup of tea or coffee but sometimes they will say they will have a beer. That's the only time that we tend to drink if someone comes and they have one. Just for ourselves, we don't bother.

This comment is interesting because it is her partner who will offer the refreshment if it is alcoholic. The gender of the visitor could also affect what was offered: 'I usually offer them a drink, tea or something, or if it's a man he might have a drink rather

than tea or coffee. I offer them both and something to eat . . .
biscuits, cake, sandwich – or if we're going to have a meal I say
"Do you want to stop?".'

These 'snacks' with cups of tea and coffee were something to
be avoided for those women who were dieting, and cigarettes
were a way of avoiding eating. One woman explained her
situation:

> . . . girls round here come in and they have a coffee. [So you'd give them
> a coffee and would you give them anything else?] No because – well a
> lot of them smoke so they have a coffee and a cigarette really. I would
> offer them a biscuit or if I've baked a piece of cake or something but
> they very rarely eat because they have a cigarette.

The provision of a drink, with or without food, provides an
opportunity for a chat which would not arise if it was not
forthcoming. For some women this was very important as it
gave them a chance to talk about their problems with their
friends. One woman met her friends regularly for a coffee: she
was asked whether she found the meetings helpful:

> Definitely, because, let's face it, men don't worry so much as women do.
> I mean if a woman gets something on her mind she blows it up out of all
> proportion, doesn't she, if you're like me you do, and it's nothing really.
> But I think a lot of it is that because you are on your own so much . . . I
> mean my husband is never at home, he's always out somewhere
> gadding about but it's usually work. To me it's nice to be able to talk to
> other women and then you come home feeling loads better because you
> think, 'Well, God I'm not the only one that's got all these problems,
> they're worse than me'. I think I shouldn't get upset about odd silly
> little things because they've got it worse than me and I always come
> home feeling better.

Cake and biscuits were usually the foods that accompanied tea
or coffee, most frequently biscuits. And this use of food by
almost half the women in our sample provides an indication of
why these types of foods are eaten between meals. Offering
people food and drink and even encouraging them to forage for
themselves is all part of making them feel welcome and at home.
When it is not provided it is felt as a lack, an indication of how
welcome, or unwelcome, someone is. Its non-provision can be a
means of restricting the timespan of a visit to the minimum
necessary for its purpose.

There is a variation in the food and drink offered to a casual
visitor depending on women's occupational class; the pattern is

not so clear for men's occupational class. Women in occupational classes I/II are more likely than others to offer food to casual visitors and are more likely than other women to offer alcohol to evening visitors. In occupational classes I/II 27 (64·3%) of women offered food and a drink to daytime and evening visitors compared to 2 (28·6%) of women in occupational classes IV/V. And 2 (4·8%) of women in occupational classes I/II might offer a casual visitor an alcoholic drink during the daytime while 12 (28·6%) of them might in the evening. This compares with no-one in occupational classes IV/V offering alcohol to casual visitors.

This class difference may be explained by income differences, although if this were the whole explanation we would expect there to be a closer correlation with men's occupational class than there is. Many women mentioned that they bought fewer cakes and biscuits than they had in the past because of their cost, but the difference in the offering of alcohol ties in with the class patterns of alcohol consumption that we have already explored.

Entertaining family

Most women, when people were coming to share a meal with them, cooked or presented the food in a special way; more of an effort was made. The treatment given to their immediate families was often less elaborate than that accorded to friends, and for business friends arrangements were at their most formal. These differences reveal that as well as being a sign of welcome and hospitality, the provision of food, the type of food, the setting of the table and the way the food is served, all convey messages about the status of the visitors and the importance of their visit and, at the same time, reflect the status and living standards of the family whose home is being visited. The immediate family who visits regularly does not need to be impressed as much as a friend who is not seen very often. On the other hand, if friends arrive unexpectedly, food is not usually prepared more elaborately than usual, just asking them to join in with the meal that is already being prepared for the family makes them feel welcome.

Most of the women shared meals with their families and friends; 131 (65·5%) invited their families to their homes for meals, 117 (58·5%) invited close friends and 7 (3·5%) invited business friends to eat with them. There seem to be class differences in the frequency with which women share meals with their extended families. Working-class women are more likely to share meals with their extended family on a regular basis than are women from occupational classes I/II, while the latter do not often share meals with them unless they come to stay. In occupational classes I/II 8 (13·3%) women shared meals with members of their extended family during the week or at weekends compared with 9 (32·1%) women in class IIIN, 31 (39·7%) women in class IIIM and 8 (38·1%) women in classes IV/ V, whereas 15 (25%) women in occupational classes I/II shared meals with their extended family when they came to stay. The figures for the other occupational classes are: IIIN 0, IIIM 5 (6·4%), IV/V 2 (9·5%). This difference between the classes can largely be explained by the fact that women in occupational classes I/II are likely to live some distance away from their parents which means that coming together for a meal is not practicable. So the only time they eat together is when they stay in each other's houses. Women in the other occupational classes were much more likely to live at least in the same town as their parents and so coming round for a meal was easy.

Sunday seemed to be the day that was set aside for sharing meals with the extended family. Women would either go to their parents' or parents'-in-law for Sunday 'dinner' or, frequently, they invited their parents and other members of their families round for tea. This often involved them in more elaborate preparation than usual: 'I would try to make it a bit nicer – get extra things for the salad, do an extra cake or something else special like that. I get out the best cloth and use the best cutlery. I use the tea set and get out nicer dishes than every day.' Inviting the family to tea on Sunday could be quite a regular occurrence: 'My husband's sister and her husband come for Sunday tea every other week. When Gordon's on 2 to 10 I sometimes have my friend round from work to tea. My mother sometimes comes to tea.' Sunday was clearly a family day, more so in households where the extended family lived close together than in others, and this pattern was more common amongst working-class households. This regularity of contact between family members seemed to reduce the need women felt to provide something out of the ordinary for their visitors. Although it might be felt necessary to impress parents-in-law more than parents, as this woman told us. If her parents came round the food would be: 'The same as what we're having. If Dave's parents come round we make something a bit different. They usually come for tea – they're good cooks so I feel a bit embarrassed having them for dinner – I do a buffet, have a good spread.'

Women in occupational classes I/II were more likely to cook something special, serve it in a way that was different from normal, and provide alcohol with the meal than were other women. Thus, 43·3% of women in classes I/II always cooked something special for family guests compared with 24% of women in class IIIN, 20·6% of women in class IIIM and 16·7% of women in classes IV and V. The differences in presenting food in a special way were even greater, with 60·6% of women in classes I/II doing this for family guests compared with 32·5% of women in class IIIN, 25% of women in class IIIM and 18·2% of women in classes IV and V. Similarly, alcohol was served by 33·3% of women in classes I/II, 16·9% of women in class IIIN, 20% of women in class IIIM and 9·1% of women in classes IV and V. These differences can probably be seen as resulting from the infrequency with which class I/II households shared meals as an extended family. For them it was a special occasion, something out of the ordinary, whereas for women whose parents lived 'up the road' it was much more likely to be a normal part of daily family life. The difference in the provision of alcohol ties in with all our findings on alcohol, but also reflects the type of meal that was shared with the extended family. It would not be appropriate in any household to serve alcohol with Sunday tea, but with an evening meal or a Sunday 'dinner' it might be.

The message of welcome that is encoded in food and drink and the way it is presented is usually read unconsciously, and it is only when it is missing that we become aware of the meanings carried by meals and their provision. One woman told us at length what happened when she went to visit her parents-in-law, and her story brings out clearly the importance of food to social relations:

When he [partner] talks of being at home he always talks of when . . . you see his mum and dad, his first dad I should say and his mum, were

divorced. He always seems to talk of before they were divorced when it
was like a happy family and he can remember when his mum used to
make these gorgeous chocolate cakes. It sounds very nice but he never
seems to talk about what went wrong you see. I've only ever known
them when the meals have been terrible. To me they are nothing to fill
you at all. The times that Bob and I have been to stay we've been
permanently starving. I'm not kidding, we've gone there, it's not very
often we go 'cos I've got so fed up with it although I know occasionally
we do have to go. We go about once a year or once every two years,
something like that. But it has been a total disappointment. We used to
set off after having a slice of toast each . . . and we've got there about 11
o'clock and you've been given a coffee. As soon as you get in you
definitely get a coffee. So we've had a coffee by 12 – half past 12 they go
to the pub so you're left sat there if you don't want to go. There's no
organisation at all in the house – you're just left sat there. They come
back and about 3 o'clock they politely ask if you want a sandwich. Now
to me, especially when you have got such a . . . it gets beyond a joke.
And then it's been time to come home. Or she's decided about 3 o'clock
suddenly you can have a cooked meal and I always remember one of
them was a pork chop, and really green, oh, it was really irony – I've
never had one so irony in all my life – cabbage, and a couple of new
potatoes. Now that to me is – I mean if you've gone anywhere you
usually make an effort. When I do have family coming there is more of
an effort made than there is normally. I mean they're given notice that
you're coming and I said to Bob, 'You'd imagine that she would have
had a meal waiting and ready', but no . . . Well, the last time I went, it
would have been nearly 2 years ago going by Eva's age, we got there
abut 11, coffee, sister Sue was there and husband and little boy.
'Where's mum?' 'Oh, she's got a migraine, she's in bed.' Well, I said to
Bob that she could have 'phoned us and cancelled it. So Bob had his
audience with mum upstairs – I'm sat downstairs for about an hour.
Down he came and then 'it's your turn to go up, take the children'. So I
went up and she said 'I'm going to get up, I'm going to get up'. I went
downstairs and waited another hour for her to come down. Then it was
pub time, so off to the pub. She stayed at home and when we got back
from there there was nothing, nothing to eat or anything. I said to Bob
that that was the last time I went. Even when his Dad died I didn't go to
the funeral. I said to Bob that after church 'You know where you'll be –
at the pub, I'm not going, what do I do with Robert? No, I'm not going.' I
didn't go and it was a pub do. Like my mum said at the time, that it was
just unbelievable, you know, when I told her the things we'd gone there
and had. I mean we have been a couple of times when his mum and dad
were in France and there was just Sue and her husband. She is worse
than mum. You arrive there and you can hear them about four hours
after you've got there – they're in the kitchen – 'What are we going to
give them?' 'I don't know, what you got?' They come through, 'Do you
fancy corned beef or cheese?' and that's how it is. It irritates me to
think that when they come everything's done that bit special. Well, I

consider it is when you go out of your way to get something special for them.

She later told us about the effort she makes when she has any member of her family visiting:

They usually just ring up and say when they're coming and I say 'For dinner or dinner and tea?' and we sort it out like that. [But do you cook anything special?] If they're coming for dinner I usually do a roast dinner, even if it's in the middle of the week. I find it is easier, I'll do a roast dinner. If it's for tea or it's a hot day or anything like that I often get a ham joint and do that and do new potatoes and salad. [And what would you have for drink?] Well, if it's with a dinner, if it's at dinner time, we usually buy a bottle of wine – if my mum or my sister comes we buy a bottle of wine to have with the dinner. But if it's just for tea it's usually just a pot of tea. Bob and I will more often drink coffee but my family drink more tea and the teapot comes out.

Clearly, for her the inability to provide food appropriate to a family visit, in some fundamental way signalled the breakdown of the social relations constituting the family. This breakdown and its repercussions in food provision underline the importance of food in maintaining and reproducing social, in this case familial, cohesion.

Whereas sharing meals with the extended family, an event which almost by definition included children, was least common amongst occupational class I/II women, entertaining and being entertained by friends was most common. This can be seen in Table 9.10.

Table 9.10 *Patterns of entertainment by women's social class, (n = 195) – no. (%) (Percentages do not always total 100)*

	I/II	IIIN	IIIM	IV/V	Student	Total
Family only	2 (4·8)	26 (25·0)	11 (37·9)	7 (38·9)	–	46 (23·6)
Friends only	12 (28·6)	14 (13·5)	5 (17·2)	3 (16·7)	1 (50·0)	35 (17·9)
Family and friends	25 (59·5)	42 (40·4)	6 (20·7)	3 (16·7)	1 (50·0)	77 (39·5)
Friends and business friends	–	2 (1·9)	1 (3·4)	–	–	3 (1·5)
All	1 (2·4)	3 (2·9)	–	–	–	4 (2·1)
No one	1 (2·4)	16 (15·4)	6 (20·7)	5 (27·8)	–	28 (14·4)
Other	1 (2·4)	1 (1·0)	–	–	–	2 (1·0)
Total	42 (100·0)	104 (100·0)	29 (100·0)	18 (100·0)	2 (100·0)	195 (100·0)

This shows that family entertaining becomes more common as we move from social classes I and II to social classes IV and V, and entertaining family and friends and friends alone become less common. Women in classes I and II are more likely to entertain friends than those in any other social group. It also shows that women in occupational classes IV/V are less likely than those in the other classes to invite anyone to eat in their homes whereas occupational class I/II women are most likely to.

Meals that were cooked for friends were almost always more elaborate than ordinary family meals and also differed from those that might be shared with the extended family. This is both a display of a family's status and a welcome for and way of respecting and acknowledging the status of visitors. One woman explained how meals for friends differed from daily cooking for the family.

I usually consult my cookery books then and try to find something new for a change . . . I like to put a nice table cloth on the table and we use the good plates. I don't put candles on the table. I used to when I was first married. That must have been when I was drunk with the idea of having my own home.

So it was not only the food that was special but also the way the table was set out and the way the food was served. Everything was 'dressed up' a bit and special food was bought; the appearance of food becomes much more important when friends have been invited to share it.

I love entertaining, 'cos as I say, as I've told you before, I like titivating and making things look nice so I really enjoy entertaining . . . we had pheasant, I used to like doing that you see. I used to put orange twists on the top and titivate – we have big oval plates you see and if there were six of us I used to do three plates and a couple got a plate between them and I used to chop the pheasant in half and then put all the trimmings round it.

But entertaining in this way was also more expensive than normal, family eating, especially if special, high status foods were bought, which they usually were. In fact, 90 (45%) of the women who entertained friends always cooked something out of the ordinary for them compared to 13 (6·5%) who sometimes did and 19 (9·5%) who cooked as they would have normally. The proportion of women cooking special food for visiting family members was much lower. A high proportion of women also presented and served the food differently from the way they normally did. One woman told us the sort of changes she made. 'I serve it out in the kitchen unless we have anyone come in when I'll put it in dishes and put it on the table.'

There did not seem to be any clear class pattern in the preparation of special food and its more elaborate presentation. Women throughout the class structure gave their friends this special treatment. However, what did vary with class was whether alcohol was drunk with the meal. Thus 71·8% of women in occupational classes I/II always gave their friends alcohol with a meal compared with 61·3% of women in class IIIN, 45·4% of women in class IIIM and 50% of women in classes IV and V. Conversely, only 5·1% of women in classes I/II never served alcohol with a meal they were sharing with friends, compared with just over 16% of women in classes IIIN, IV and V and 27·2% of women in class IIIM.

The provision of elaborate meals consisting of high-status foods is a way of impressing as well as making people feel welcome. Women often voiced the pressure they felt they were under which, for some of them, made the experience of cooking for visitors nerve-racking, and led others to abandon formal entertaining altogether. Cooking a meal for visitors is, in some way, a presentation of status and skills to the outside world and women and their families are judged on the basis of what they provide.

Some women were confident about their ability to impress:

Dinner parties even now – if I'm – I suppose it's just a way of – if I'm cooking something I'm good at – that sounds faintly modest but there's no point lying about it – because I like it I suppose I'm good at it and because I'm good at it I like it and I still try to impress people with it, colleagues and things of Tony's so there it is . . . it's so calculated. You've got to admit to going out of your way to doing something.

But others got very nervous and found it something of an ordeal:

I just had no confidence that I would be able to produce anything reasonable anyway, so I didn't [cook]. I was very badly brought up, you see, not being forced to learn anything useful . . . I forced myself to learn because I wanted to have people round for meals and in London especially, if you wanted to see people in the evening they would have to eat with you. So that's what pushed me into learning to cook so that occasionally I could entertain my friends . . . that pushed me into at least making an attempt but I was terribly nervous.

Women, food and families

In a slightly different context one of the women put her finger on an important reason for this anxiety about cooking for other people. It is often the only form of intervention in the outside world for women who are at home all day with young children:

Like the kitchen was my form of expression. Cake making was my form of expression . . . I don't do it now but food was obviously being – there was some function being offered to food. Something to do with some sort of sense of social inadequacy or lack of self-awareness . . . I don't do it any more and that might be because I'm better expressed in the work I'm doing than I was then.

Cooking, in these circumstances, is a representation of a woman's worth, if she does it well she is judged to be not only a good cook but also a good wife and mother, if she does not do it well she is failing in her allotted feminine role. For women who have no means of acquiring self-confidence and self-esteem through employment outside the home, cooking and, in particular, entertaining become a means of representing her talents as well as the status of the family. One woman spoke about this:

Dave thinks I'm a good cook but I don't think I am particularly, so I don't like cooking for people, I feel awkward at the table when I've dished something up and they all say 'Oh, this is delicious', and I always think 'Oh, they don't really like it', you know, and I'm sort of making excuses all the time saying 'it's not as good as it usually is' . . . but everybody always thinks it's quite nice, but I just don't like doing it, I find it embarrassing.

This fear of failure leads some women to cook only familiar dishes if friends are coming for a meal: 'If somebody's coming it's easier for me to do something terribly basic like a chicken casserole, it's easier to do something that I know I can cook well rather than trying something different that might not turn out at all.'

A way of avoiding this judgmental aspect of entertaining and yet still sharing meals with friends was to encourage them to stay for meals if they called round for a visit. One woman said: 'They turn up more or less at the door and I say "Do you want to stop 'cos I'm cooking already?" It's not often I make arrangements for people to come down because as I say I don't like cooking for people very much, I'd rather go out for a meal with them.' It is clear that an impromptu meal such as this cannot be compared to a meal which has been arranged in advance and therefore the judgmental aspect is removed; what is then dominant is hospitality, readiness to offer food to visitors even when they drop in unannounced.

On the other hand, many women said that they really enjoyed entertaining, and certainly preferred cooking something special for friends to cooking the daily round of family meals:

I don't enjoy cooking every day ... if I was inviting a couple of friends round I would enjoy doing a meal ... but I don't enjoy thinking, 'Oh, he's coming home, what the hell can I give him tonight?' – that is a bit of a bore – but I don't dislike cooking.

It was almost always women who cooked for friends: in fact in only three households did the man cook, in nine the cooking was shared and in a further seven either partner might cook.

In those families where the man cooked it was usually his only contribution to the family's cuisine and he only engaged in this more elaborate cooking for visitors; the daily round of family cooking was, virtually without exception, left to the women:

He likes to bake, he likes baking and he likes doing fancy stuff. He's not so keen on doing plain things, he finds that boring, he likes all the fancy stuff ... if we're having a dinner party then he'll cook that, he likes doing that sort of thing ... he'll sort of go through the cookery books and pick out a main meal, he's quite good at that, he's quite good at organising it all ... Well, when we lived in Sheffield we had a couple of friends and her husband also liked to cook and they used to plan it all. They'd do the menu and then go and shop for it all, cook it, we never did a thing, it was lovely. That was when we were first married and he's always quite liked to do it on occasions if we have people for dinner. [So does he go off and shop for it?] Not now, usually if he's doing it he'll say, 'Can you get such and such?', but he'll usually perhaps prepare it all, it's nice.

It was less unusual, however, for partners to help the women with meal preparation, although this still only occurred in a very small proportion of the families:

I suppose sometimes if we have someone coming for a meal he would probably – he wouldn't actually do it all but he'd do some of it ... He likes fiddling about with things, he likes experimenting with things – not to any great degree 'cos I don't like things messed about too much ... I mean when I say experiment I don't mean anything elaborate.

Because of the element of display that is involved in entertaining and the felt need to provide two or three courses of high status food in an agreeable setting, cost and lack of space both militated against women inviting their friends round for meals. One woman was living in a very small flat at the time of interview and spoke longingly of the time when she would move into a large house and have enough space to entertain. Others told similar stories. One was asked if she had friends round to eat and said: 'No, not often because as I say we haven't got room. We have friends round and if we're eating they'll eat with us and it's pot luck.' Another woman commented on the frequency of entertaining friends, she was asked how often people came for meals: 'Not as often as I would like, 'cos it is expensive, by the time you've bought the wine and everything . . . a few times a year.' Clearly, for families living on low incomes this type of entertaining is not a realistic proposition, and the inability to invite friends round and share food with them was often felt as a real deprivation.

For other families, however, sharing meals with friends was cheaper than going out for a meal with them and this had led them to invite friends round for meals whereas previously they might have eaten out together in a restaurant:

That's what we do mostly, I think. We have people here and we go to other people's houses for meals. In fact, I think I'd rather do that than go to a restaurant – particularly with a couple of friends, sometimes we say, 'Let's buy some food in and we'll cook a meal', we do that. I think you can cook a better meal and it costs a lot less, yes, so I suppose the money side of it does come into it there.

Several women commented on the problems of combining entertaining with having young children:

We don't have people as often for a meal now as I would like to. There's a lot of friends I'm wanting to say 'Come for a meal one evening' but because of the children we don't commit ourselves yet because I think it spoils the evening 'cos they're usually pretty good at going to bed, but Joanne, if she's teething, you might just get her off to sleep and at 9 o'clock you're bringing her down. If I'm busy cooking, sort of entertaining, then it spoils it, so I think well, I'd rather not bother at the moment.

This problem could be avoided by inviting friends to tea, or Sunday dinner, particularly if they had children of their own, and in this case the type of food laid on was akin to that enjoyed by family visitors:

If they are going to come round it's usually for Sunday dinner because with not having a very large house it makes it difficult on an evening really and, you know, you're so taken up with putting the kids to bed and having her as well. I think that maybe when she's a bit older then we are – we have plans for a big kitchen on the back and that will be the boy's bedroom. I think I'll have more evening meals then, but at the moment they just join in the family meal.

Clearly, having children placed restraints on evening entertaining and it was easier to invite friends and their children, or family members, round to share in a family meal rather than preparing and cooking a special meal in the evening. When entertaining family members the meal was likely to be shared by the extended family, including children, and often took the form of a proper, family 'dinner' or 'tea'. However, children were much less likely to be present at mealtimes when friends were sharing the meal; they had normally been put to bed by the time the guests arrived. This restriction of a shared meal to adult friends, and the provision of high status food and drink which is often viewed as inappropriate for children and can be expensive, helps to explain why some women felt unable to entertain friends while their children were so young. This type of meal is for adults only, 'adult' food and drink are consumed and children are not expected to be present or to make their presence felt. Women, rather than breaking with these conventions, retire from these social gatherings for as long as their children are likely to interrupt the proceedings or even insist on being present. In all occupational classes it was more likely that children would be excluded from this type of meal which contrasts with meals shared with members of the extended family when children were normally present. However, it is most likely that children whose mothers are in occupational classes I/II will be excluded. In 19 (45·2%) families with women in classes I/II, children were not present at this type of meal, compared with 29 (27·9%) in class IIIN, 4 (13·8%) in class IIIM and 5 (27·8%) in classes IV/V.

The serving of alcohol at meals that friends were sharing was a task which was often allocated to the man, and again the gender division seemed to be clearer in working-class than middle-class families. For instance, the partners of 18 (46·1%) of women in occupational classes I/II served alcohol to visitors while in occupational class IIIN 31 (54·5%) of men did, in occupational class IIIM 6 (66·7%) of the men did and in occupational classes IV/V 5 (100%) of the women's partners did. Serving alcohol is clearly considered to be an appropriate masculine task whereas serving other sorts of refreshment is not. One woman said: 'He'd pour it. If anybody's here for a meal he's the perfect host.' She then told us that he would never offer visitors coffee or tea:

He might carry coffee through if nobody is here – if we're on our own, he's not too bad at that. If somebody is here he won't lift a finger, I don't know why. He just doesn't like anybody to think he's under the thumb . . . he thinks it's sissy, I'm sure it's that.

Women sharing food

As well as inviting family and friends round for meals that were shared as families or as couples, some women shared meals with their women friends. These meals were usually non-main meals during the week rather than family meals on Sundays or main meals.

This type of meal, rather than reinforcing the family or displaying its status through the type of food prepared and the culinary skills of the woman, provides an opportunity for women to spend some time with each other. The provision of food and its sharing allow women to be together away from men. It is perhaps an indication of the relative weakness of these friendships between women at this stage in the life cycle that this type of meal was not frequently reported and occurred much less often than either meals with the extended family or meals as a couple with other couples. Indeed, only 28 (14%) of the women reported sharing meals with their women friends and only 5 (2·5%) said that it occurred with any regularity. Social contact between women who are mothers of young children is not encouraged within British culture. Sharing food with friends or family was most frequently undertaken as a couple or as a nuclear family. It is therefore these social relations which are reinforced through the sharing of food while those between women are not. (See D. Spender's *Man Made Language* for a similar point about space and places available for women to talk to other women (Spender, 1985: 107–8).) In addition it can be said that the social relations that women enter into outside the nuclear family are, to a large extent, mediated by their partners. They thus constitute a material representation of women's dependence on men, or at least their joint existence as a couple which forms the basis for the nuclear family. The patterns of entertaining entered into by the families in our sample seem to reinforce the couple and through it the family, in both its extended and nuclear forms, rather than any other social relationships. Additionally the class differences in patterns of entertaining are significant insofar as it is more common to share meals as an extended family within the working-class and more common to share them with friends amongst the middle class.

Meals shared by the extended family differ from those shared by friends in that they take the form of a proper family meal, usually consisting of high status meat and puddings or a proper Sunday tea. They are also suitable for children to share. Meals for friends, however, usually consist of 'adult' food and drink, food cooked in alcohol for instance, or with a lot of cream, which is not considered suitable for children and which is eaten by adults only after children have gone to bed. Within the working-class, therefore, shared meals reinforce the extended family and cement links across generations, within middle-class families shared meals accentuate the divisions between adults and children in an extremely clear way; children do not share in these meals.

The class differences are significant as far as the maintenance of the extended family is concerned as it would seem that its reproduction, through the sharing of family meals, is more widespread within working-class families than amongst middle-class families where this type of sharing usually only occurs at Christmas. For middle-class families patterns of entertainment and the food consumed are different. They are more formal and elaborate and involve social relations linking adults as couples rather than adults and children as part of the extended family. This is reflected in the form of the food presented which is less often akin to a proper family meal and involves more high status ingredients and complicated preparations.

Food and drink are extremely important both as signals of hospitality and as reflections of a family's status. The food and drink which enjoy high status within British culture are typically joints of meat and steak, food that involves elaborate

and complicated preparation and contains high status ingredients such as cream or alcohol, and cream and alcohol
themselves. Meals which consist of high status ingredients are
usually more elaborately structured than ordinary family meals
having more courses and a greater choice of dishes for each
course. Often this elaboration extends to the presentation of
food and the setting of the table. Entertaining in this way
involves expense and also a lot of time; thus lack of money and
young children both militate against sharing food with visitors
in this way. The ability to do so displays a certain amount of
affluence and is a material demonstration of a family's status.

Class, gender and generational divisions are therefore reflected in and reproduced by the patterns of entertaining and in
patterns of food consumption. Thus it can be argued that
practices at the level of the provision of food and drink within
the family are determined by, and in turn reproduce, social and
sexual divisions of labour.

10
Conclusions

At the beginning of the book we said that one of our central questions was the way in which food practices contribute to the reproduction of the social order. In this chapter we wish to assess our findings in the light of this central concern, and to draw out their theoretical and practical implications.

Throughout we have focused our discussion on three main areas, the family, women and class, and have tried to explore the way food and food practices within families with young children reflect social divisions of class, age and gender. We have argued that the food that is eaten and the form in which it is eaten convey messages about the social status of the consumers of that food, and about the social relations within which that consumption is taking place. This is not only true for relations within the family but also for relations between families. Our conclusions can therefore be divided into three separable but linked areas. Firstly, we will discuss the way that food practices reproduce the patriarchal family, characterised by the authority of the father and the subordination of the mother and, at the same time, the authority of both over the children; secondly, the particular, and often problematic, relationship women have with food which arises as a result of the gender division of labour within the family; and thirdly, the way that food practices vary across the class structure so reflecting not only patriarchal but also class divisions. Indeed, an important strand to our argument is that the form taken by the family and, particularly, the way gender divisions within it are experienced, are shaped, if not largely determined, by class.

We begin, then, by looking at the importance of food and family eating patterns for the maintenance and reproduction of the patriarchal family. Our material shows that for most of the women the regular consumption of proper meals is considered to be an important part of family life because, on the one hand, they feel it ensures that the family is eating adequately in terms of nutrition and health and, on the other hand, it demonstrates that the family is behaving in the way that families are supposed to within British culture; that is, sitting down together to share the main meal of the day. An inability to provide a proper meal, experienced particularly acutely by women managing on state benefits and low incomes, was felt to be a real deprivation, not only because they viewed it as an indication that they were unable to feed their families 'properly', but also because in some way this inability reflected on the status of their family as a 'proper' family. The provision of a proper meal seems therefore to symbolise the family. This symbolic significance is partly reflected in the way the proper meal was defined by the women we spoke to. They defined it in terms of the familiar meat (or fish) and two veg. But this was not all. A proper meal was also defined by the social relations within which it was consumed. Thus, for a meal to be proper, or even for a meat and two veg meal to be provided, all family members had to be present to consume it. That is the mother, father, and children had to eat this meal together. In addition to this it was felt that a proper meal could only be cooked by a woman. Thus the proper meal needed, for its existence, the presence of the family and, conversely, the absence of this family (e.g. if the father was away) often led to the abandonment of proper meals.

The argument that the proper meal symbolises the family implies that the relations of power which characterise the family are reproduced through its provision and consumption and this, indeed, seems to be the case. Men's authority over women and children finds representation in the selection of the food that makes up the proper meal, it usually conforms to his tastes, and in the importance attached to the provision of proper meals for men. Children learn of their father's superior authority along with the food they eat. *Their* choice is curbed and subordinated to *his* preferences at the main meal of the day while at other meals, where he is more often than not absent, they may have more choice and are often freer to take or leave the food that is available in a way that they are not if food is given to them in the form of a proper meal.

Sunday 'dinner', the proper meal par excellence, is also felt to be an important part of 'proper' family life. Consisting of roast meat, roast potatoes and fresh vegetables it was regularly eaten by almost all the families we spoke to. Again, its provision requires that all members of the family are present to eat it together.

Both the everyday proper meal and Sunday dinner are essentially 'family' meals and their consumption takes place regularly throughout the class structure, at least in families with young children. The fact that they are regarded as 'family' meals indicates that their provision and consumption are important in constituting families as 'proper' families. Their consumption holds symbolic significance for the continuance of family life. In addition, the common experience of proper meals and Sunday dinners as part of 'proper' family life, an experience which cuts across class divisions, contributes not only to the cohesion and continued existence of the family, but also to the reproduction of familial ideology. Through the provision of these meals women are confirmed in their ideologically defined position as homemakers and providers of food for others; their subordinate position in relation to men within the family is reproduced on a daily basis. Thus daily food practices within the family, because they at one and the same time reflect *and* owe their existence to social divisions of gender and age, also contribute to the reproduction of those divisions.

Christmas dinner is the prototype of the proper meal and is also, fundamentally, a celebration of the family. At Christmas time, however, it is the extended rather than the nuclear family that comes together and shares in the special food and drink. Thus as the proper meal and Sunday dinner reinforce and reproduce the nuclear family, Christmas dinner reinforces the extended family.

Divisions of gender and age are not only symbolised in the form taken by meals but are also reflected in the food that is consumed. Thus men's high status in relation to women and children is reflected in the greater consumption of foods of high status, particularly meat and alcohol, while children's status is reflected in their high consumption of low status, 'children's' food. Women's food consumption occupies an intermediate place between that of men and children, reflecting, we would argue, their power and status in relation to their children but their lack of power and status in relation to their male partners.

Food, therefore, both in the form in which it is consumed and in its distribution between members of families, reflects the social divisions of gender and age which characterise the patriarchal family. And these divisions are reproduced throughout the class structure partly through the practices surrounding the daily provision and consumption of food within the family.

Divisions of age and the passage through the different stages of childhood to adulthood are also marked by the food and drink we consume. Birthday celebrations show this most clearly as birthday food changes with a child's advance towards adulthood. But adult status is also marked by the consumption of more high status foods, such as high status meat and alcohol. The food used to mark the passing of the years in the form of birthday parties and birthday cakes shows a marked similarity throughout the class structure. And almost universally children's birthdays are regarded as important in ways that adults' are not. This is reflected in the minority of adults, particularly women, who had birthday cakes compared with the almost universal provision of birthday cakes for all except the very youngest children.

In ways such as these the food that is eaten by families reflects the social divisions which characterise them. The authority of the father is symbolised in the provision of the proper meal and the food that goes to make it up and his high status is reflected in the status of the food he eats. Similarly the lesser authority of women is reflected in their provision of proper meals *for* men and children, while children, at least at the proper meal, have to kowtow to the adults' authority, particularly their fathers', and eat what is provided. The provision of proper meals, on a daily, weekly and annual basis, symbolises and ensures the continued existence of the patriarchal family, in both its nuclear and extended form, throughout the class structure. And this provision is part of the material reality of everyday life in which familial ideology is embedded and through which it is reproduced.

The second area of concern is the relation that women have to food which arises, we have argued, from the gender division of labour within the family. Almost all the women we spoke to were responsible for the provision of food for their families. This meant that they shopped for it, cooked it and cleared away after it had been eaten. In some families men and/or children helped, but this is precisely how it was regarded, as help: the responsibility of seeing that families were fed lay wholly with women. Thus the gender division of labour conformed to the patriarchal family structure with men as the breadwinners and women as, primarily, the homemakers, although some were also in paid employment. This, however, made little difference to their responsibility for food provision. The gender division of labour therefore defines women as the servers and providers of food within the family, and they serve and provide it for men and for children. In relation to men food was regarded and used as a way of 'treating' them, expressing love and affection in the provision of special food or meals for them and in the daily provision of food that women know men will like and appreciate. In this process women's own tastes and preferences are subordinated and those of men are privileged. Indeed, it can be argued that women at this stage of the family cycle, when they are at home with small children and often financially dependent on men, feel it essential to provide men with food that they like so as to ensure their continued presence and financial support.

Food is also important in the relation between women and children and here the power lies with the women. Women feel they have to teach their children to eat 'properly' and this means eating a proper meal in a socially acceptable way. Children learn about parental authority in this way as well as about the differential power and authority exercised by their parents. They also *rebel* against this authority, and conflict at mealtimes is often a result of the process of socialisation of children that is called learning to eat properly. Women, thus, *control* their children's food intake in the interests of their healthy growth and development and the social acceptability of their behaviour. Food, particularly sweet foods, can also be used as a means of controlling children's behaviour, it can be used as a bribe or reward or withheld as punishment for unacceptable behaviour. In this process children learn not only that food satisfies hunger, but that food is a relief of boredom, a substitute for attention, a comfort when other comforts fail. Women's control over their children's food intake can be undermined by fathers and by grandparents, and they seem freer than mothers to 'treat' children with food. This is because, unlike mothers, they do not have the worry of ensuring that children eat 'properly' on a day to day basis.

This concern with children's eating extends to other members of the family, indeed women's position as servers and providers of food means that they are also concerned to keep their families fed properly and, therefore, healthily. That is, they are concerned with everyone's health except their own just as their own food preferences are the ones that are neglected.

Regular provision of proper meals for their partners and children was the way women interpreted healthy eating: thus health and nutrition were understood by means of social categories. However, although women felt *responsible* for their families' health and felt that the food eaten was important to the maintenance of health, the *control* over the food eaten by the family often lay with men. If men disliked wholemeal bread, for instance, it was not bought even if women felt it was important for nutritional and health reasons. But healthy eating was, almost universally, understood as eating properly, and this was, by definition, ensured by the regular consumption of proper meals.

Women, then, cooked proper meals for men and children regularly and liked to give pleasure to them by providing them with food they enjoyed. Indeed, the greatest pleasure in cooking lay in the relish with which it was consumed by others. This constant concern with food and its centrality to the role of wife and mother sat ill with an equally strongly felt need to control women's own food intake in the interest of maintaining sexual attractiveness and retaining partners' affection. Food for most women was at the same time an enemy and a friend. An enemy because eating it led to an unwanted increase in weight, a friend because food is often turned to as a comfort in times of stress and as a relief from boredom – a lesson that is learnt in childhood. So while women are feeding men and children wholesome, nourishing food, they are denying it to themselves in the interests of maintaining a usually unnaturally slim body image. Women's widespread dissatisfaction with their own weight did not affect their families' food intake nor the women's concern over the weight and health of their partners and children. Indeed, while concern over their own weight was almost entirely due to dissatisfaction with their appearance, concern over men's and children's weight was much more often linked to concern over the health implications of obesity. This double standard links to ideologies of sexuality and food needs and is related to the supposed 'natural' differences between men and women that automatically lead to men having bigger appetites, because they are physically bigger and 'need' more energy than women. This differentiation of food needs along lines of gender begins at puberty and leads to girls 'naturally' wanting to slim and remain pre-pubertal in shape and boys 'naturally' indulging in activities which require lots of energy and wanting to grow and become 'big', 'strong' men.

The gender division of labour which characterises the patriarchal family therefore has profound implications for women's relationship to food. Familial ideology, which defines man as breadwinner and woman as homemaker, coexists with ideologies of sexuality and ideological evaluations of men's and women's work. This combination results in a dual standard which permits men a larger body size than women and enables them to intervene effectively in the outside world. Women, as sexual ornaments and as 'non-participants' in the world of work, are condemned to a permanent struggle against food. This struggle produces an illusion of control and has the effect of deflecting their potential for meaningful intervention in the world of men. Thus, women are centrally concerned with food, they are with it all day and every day, they feed others and give others pleasure through food, yet they deny it to themselves in the interest of maintaining an alluring figure, because food is short and others' needs take precedence over their own and because concern to satisfy others' likes and dislikes leads to a total submerging of their own preferences.

Our third focus is on the way class divisions are reflected in food practices and the way class affects diet. Class differences in the food eaten by families and in the way it is eaten are largely a result of material circumstances although ideology, specifically food ideologies, also has a part to play. Fundamentally, however, it is the material circumstances of people's lives which give rise to class differences in family food practices. The material circumstances to which we are referring include factors such as the level of income, housing, employment and unemployment, hours of work and whether or not families live near their parents or parents-in-law. Through its impact on these factors, class affects the food eaten, meal patterns, food ideologies, ideas on nutrition, and patterns of hospitality and entertaining. It also shapes the form taken by the patriarchal family and the way in which gender divisions are lived.

Class, through its effect on income, affects the food that women can afford to buy. Thus although women in all social classes felt a proper meal was important and food was crucial to the maintenance of health, working-class women managing on low incomes were less able to put these ideas into practice than middle-class women whose food buying was not so constrained by considerations of expense. Thus managing on a low income meant that considerations of cost took precedence over considerations of the nutritional value of food and this partly explains some of the observed class differences in food consumption. As we all know, if the diet is constructed around the provision of a meat and two veg meal, then to eat nutritious food and food that is *socially* valued is often more expensive than to buy food which is less 'good' for you. We only have to think of the cost of a white sliced loaf compared with a wholemeal loaf or sausages in comparison with beef to realise the constraints placed upon families' diets by low income.

This, of course, assumes that the food eaten and valued conforms to the dominant food ideology. 'Alternative' food ideologies, such as vegetarianism, were totally confined to middle-class women; but their wider existence could moderate the effect of income on diet and cheaper food would then be substituted for meat and the proper meal may altogether be abandoned. However, across the class structure the majority of women constructed their families' diets around the proper meal, which almost always had meat as its central element. And given this adherence to the dominant food ideology, income had a marked effect on diet.

Similarly most women, whatever their class, preferred the main meal to be eaten at the table together as a family.

However, a lack of space in working-class homes often meant that this ideal was unattainable. Middle-class homes were much more likely to have space in the kitchen or a dining room in which to eat. So in this way class affects whether or not meals are eaten at table. It seemed also that main meals tended to be more formal in middle-class than working-class families. They were more likely to be at table, talking was encouraged and the television and radio were less likely to be on. Thus the *experience* of family eating, even though the proper meal and Sunday dinner were universally regarded as important to family life, and were almost universally provided, differed according to class.

However, the timing of the main meal almost universally depended on when the male partner could be home from work, and women in all social classes are past-mistresses at denying themselves and meeting the needs of others. Thus gender divisions exist throughout the class structure. The almost universal privileging of men's food preferences by women means that men largely control families' diets, and it also means that men's preferences influence *class* differences in diet. However, while these aspects of the gender division of labour may be apparent throughout the class structure there are others which vary with class. For instance there seemed to be a tendency towards more 'sharing' and gender 'equality' within middle-class families than working-class families. Thus, money management and shopping for food were more likely to be shared by middle-class marriage partners while the gender division of labour was more clearly demarcated within the working class with women usually shopping on their own. Similarly, whether alcohol was drunk by men in the pub or by men and women at home together depended on class; the former being more likely within working-class families. And in middle-class families, although there seemed to be less clearly defined spheres of activity for men and women which, apparently, produced more 'sharing', gender inequality persisted in other forms. Having said that, however, where income was low, and particularly where men were unemployed, there seemed to be less gender inequality, at least in terms of the frequency of food consumption, than in any other situation. And the families where this was the case were all working class. Thus the inequalities arising from the gender division of labour may partly be a result of the 'fact' that men as the breadwinners need to be fed and looked after to a greater extent than any other member of the family, precisely because their continued ability to go out to work is crucial for the support of the family. Male unemployment changes this situation and affects gender inequality in terms of food consumption.

Patterns of hospitality and entertaining are also affected by class. Within the working class meals are more likely to be shared by members of the extended family on a regular basis than they are in middle-class families; whereas 'dinner parties' for adults only are the most common form of entertaining with food amongst middle-class families. This difference can partly be explained by the greater likelihood of middle-class women and men living some distance away from their parents and siblings. This also explains why Christmas dinner is often the only time middle-class extended families share food together. Additionally, entertaining with food is an expensive business and requires space, two factors clearly militating against women on low incomes attempting it at all.

Sharing food with others was, throughout the class structure, most likely to take place as a couple or a family. Women hardly ever shared a meal with friends on their own. These food practices therefore reinforce social relations constituting the couple or the family rather than any other social relations, and indicate that women's contacts with the 'outside' world largely take place within the context of the patriarchal family. Indeed women's culinary skills are often their only form of intervention in the outside world and are used to display their qualities as a 'good' wife and mother. The form taken by women's restriction within patriarchal social relations, however, varies with class. Within the working class shared meals reinforce the extended family and cement links across generations while within the middle class shared meals, in the form of dinner parties which exclude children, divide adults and children and rarely reinforce the extended family.

Divisions of age, unlike gender divisions, do not display any class variation which suggests that the ideology of childhood is strong and almost uniform throughout the class structure. However, greater indulgence towards children, specifically in the form of 'treating' with food, is more apparent within working-class families, where means permit, than within middle-class families.

Finally a large part of our argument has been that food conveys messages and indicates or reflects social relations and divisions. It is universally used as a sign of hospitality and its provision, or lack of it, is a powerful means of including or excluding people. Thus the sharing of meals by families symbolises their existence as a social entity. Food also carries social status and value and its differential consumption by men and women, adults and children, and between the classes, reflects differences in power and status which arise from the social divisions of gender, age and class. The food that is eaten, however, not only *reflects* these divisions, it also recreates them on a daily basis, and the form of this creation varies with class. This means that people in different classes have different experiences of food and family life even though familial ideology, and its material representation in the form of the proper meal, are ubiquitous. There seems to be a tendency towards more so-called 'equality' between men and women within the middle class while adult–child divisions are more marked. In contrast gender divisions seem to take the form of 'separate spheres' within working-class families while adult–child divisions are not so sharply demarcated. Most of these differences can be seen as a result of class-related differences in people's material circumstances rather than as products of 'faulty' child-rearing practices or lack of understanding of nutritional principles. However, although the precise form taken by gender and age divisions may depend on class, gender and age divisions persist throughout the class structure. Women are subordinate to men and children are subordinate to adults. And these social relations of power are reflected in every aspect of family eating that we have explored. Returning to our original question we can therefore say that food practices within the family reflect *and reproduce* social divisions of gender, age and class and, because of this, contribute to the maintenance of the social order – a social order characterised by inequalities between women and men, adults and children and different social classes.

These, then, are our main conclusions at the level of theory. The practical and policy implications of our research remain to be explored.

We said at the outset that if a general improvement in the diet of the nation is aimed for, and change in eating habits is regarded as desirable, an essential prerequisite is an understanding of the social significance and functions of food. It is important to understand why people eat what they eat and the constraints within which they operate. One of the major constraints, and one that was felt as such by many of the women, is the organisation of food production and the control exerted by food manufacturers over the kind of food that is available in the shops. Given the massive use of insecticides within agriculture, for instance, it is almost impossible to buy fruit and vegetables that are not in some way contaminated, whatever the level of nutritional knowledge of the consumer. To argue, therefore, that policies to change food habits should be aimed solely at the consumer is doomed to failure, unless pressure is also put on the producers and manufacturers to change the type of food they make available. And it could be argued that the latter course of action, particularly if it were backed by law, would have much more effect much more rapidly than the former. However, as Doyal argues for the case of the tobacco companies, too much is at stake in terms of lost profits and loss of revenue for governments managing a capitalist economy to take this course of action (Doyal, 1981). This almost fatally weakens any attempts to transform the diet and defines the problem as an individual one. Individuals can 'choose' what diet to follow and this position leads to the view put forward so clearly by Edwina Currie, among others, that people, particularly those in the North of England (our area of study) have only their own ignorance to blame for not eating a nutritious and healthy diet. As we have shown, this is by no means the whole story. Most women have some awareness of current nutritional thinking, but there are a number of practical constraints which militate against them putting these ideas into practice apart from the primary and major constraints provided by the food manufacturers and agribusiness.

Firstly, nutritional 'experts' are often seen to disagree amongst themselves and, in addition, there seem to be 'fashions' in nutritional thinking; what is 'good' for you one year is 'bad' for you the next. This situation not unnaturally leads to scepticism. Despite the scepticism and the need to take all these expert opinions 'with a pinch of salt' (although, even this may no longer be advisable) women feel responsible for the health of their families and do take into account the 'goodness' of food, if the other constraints under which they operate allow. But these other constraints often mean that the construction of a diet along sound nutritional lines is a luxury that can only be indulged in by middle-class women, who are either not constrained by considerations of income or who espouse alternative food ideologies and therefore do not feel compelled to spend a large proportion of the money allocated to food on relatively expensive meat.

The constraints under which women operate if they are providing food in accordance with the dominant food ideology are many. Firstly, the provision of a proper meal is regarded as central to family life and essential to ensure that men and children are eating properly. In addition to this men are seen as deserving and needing a proper meal and meat is regarded as an essential part, particularly of men's diets. Thus, exhortations to eat more beans and pulses, even if women are willing to listen, are likely to produce meagre results because beans and pulses neither fit into the structure of the proper meal, *nor* are they highly *socially* valued within the dominant food ideology. Their lowly social status means their high nutritional status is likely to go unappreciated and untried. The centrality of the proper meal to family eating is therefore a significant constraint limiting the types of changes that can be made to the diet. Food manufacturers are acutely aware of this, convenience foods are all substitutes for elements of the proper meal and where innovation *does* occur it is most frequently in the type of food eaten between meals or at meals other than the proper meal. Witness the ever growing and changing number of breakfast cereals, crisps of an infinite variety of flavours and chocolate bars, for instance.

Secondly, women are constrained by men's food preferences and, to a much lesser extent, children's. Many men have a 'conservative' taste in food and dislike any innovation, they prefer the meat and two veg meal they've always been used to.

The need to provide food that is appreciated by men therefore militates against any innovation in the diet even when women themselves would be interested in such a change.

Income, as we have already mentioned, severely limits the nutritional status of the diet when we take into account the desire (itself socially constructed) to provide proper meals regularly and Sunday dinner once a week. This is barely possible on a low income, and if it is managed the meat in particular is likely to be the cheapest available and therefore neither highly socially valued nor with high nutritional content. Thus, exigencies of income, the centrality of the proper meal to the family, the dominance of *men's* tastes and the problems associated with feeding children which often lead women to resort to 'children's' food that they know will be eaten, all need to be taken into account if change in the diet is the aim.

Currently, nutrition education is aimed at women. We would argue that this, far from leading to a healthy transformation in families' diets actually increases the burden of guilt carried by women. This is because they are usually unable to follow or even to accept the advice that they are given because it does not fit in with the lived reality of providing food on a daily basis for their family. This was given concrete form by the women we talked to when they discussed the advice given to them by health care professionals. They often sought advice if their child would not eat, which we now understand to mean they would not eat a proper meal. They were reassured in various ways and told not to worry, their child would be getting the nutrients they needed from whatever it was they were eating. But this was not the issue and the reassurances did not help. The health care professionals missed the point entirely because they did not understand that women feel that children must learn to eat food in the form of a proper meal. *This* is the problem they present, and no amount of reassurance about the nutritional status of a child's diet will help if the child continues to refuse to eat 'properly'. An understanding of the social construction of diet and, indeed, of the social meaning of eating properly is vital in order to be able to understand, let alone solve, the problem women are facing when their child will not eat 'properly'. Their concern is over more than the nutritional status of the child's diet, it is a concern to integrate the child into the social order as it is represented within the family, and as it is symbolised in the daily provision and consumption of the proper meal.

We are arguing, therefore, that targeting women is not an adequate means of improving or changing families' diets. Targeting men and educating boys and girls in school might have slightly more impact. But transforming food ideologies and the social values attached to food might be even more effective. However, even if such a propaganda campaign were adequately funded and effective at the level of individuals' decisions about the foods they would like to buy and eat, without a simultaneous transformation in the food that is available on the supermarket shelves, the nation's diet would be extremely slow to respond. In addition, food that was nutritionally desirable would have to be marketed at prices that could be afforded by those on low incomes, and this is way outside the control of women who are struggling to feed their partners and children on an income which is barely enough to manage on.

We are arguing, therefore, that at a practical level the most effective way of influencing diet would be to control the production of food, any other strategy is far less likely to succeed. But if another strategy *is* adopted then it has to take into consideration that food is not only eaten to satisfy physiological needs and to keep body and soul together, but that the food we eat and the form that we eat it in are themselves socially constructed and meet many needs that are socially, rather than biologically, determined. Without such an understanding any attempt at successful intervention is unlikely to be effective and will only serve to increase the burden of guilt which already weighs so heavily on the shoulders of women.

Bibliography

Althusser, L. 'Ideology and ideological state apparatuses', in *Lenin and Philosophy*, NLB, 1971.

Barrett, M. *Women's Oppression Today*, Verso, 1980.

Barthes, R. 'Towards a psychosociology of contemporary food consumption', in *Food and Drink in History: Selections from the Annales Economies, Societies, Civilisations*, R. Forster and O. Ranum (eds), Johns Hopkins University Press, 1979.

Bilton, T. *et al. Introductory Sociology*, Macmillan, 1984.

Bourdieu, P. *Outline of a Theory of Practice*, Cambridge University Press, 1977.

Boyd-Orr, J. *Food, Health and Income*, Macmillan, 1936.

Burton, C. *Subordination: Feminism and Social Theory*, George Allen and Unwin, 1985.

Charles, N. and Brown, D. 'Women, shiftwork and the sexual division of labour', in *The Sociological Review*, vol. 29, no. 4, University of Keele, 1981, pp. 685–704.

Charles, N. and Kerr, M. 'Eating properly, the family and state benefit', in *Sociology*, vol. 20, no. 3, 1986a, pp. 412–419.

Charles, N. and Kerr, M. 'Issues of responsibility and control in the feeding of families', in *The Politics of Health Education*, S. Rodmell and A. Watt (eds), RKP, 1986b, pp. 57–75.

Chernin, K. *Womansize: The Tyranny of Slenderness*, Women's Press, 1983.

Chernin, K. *The Hungry Self*, Virago, 1986.

COMA (see DHSS).

Delamont, S. *The Sociology of Women*, George Allen and Unwin, 1980.

Delphy, C. 'Sharing the same table: consumption and the family', in *The Sociology of the Family: New Directions for Britain*, Chris Harris (ed.), Sociological Review Monograph 28, University of Keele, 1979.

DHSS *Diet and Cardiovascular Disease*, Report of the Committee on Medical Aspects of Food Policy (COMA), HMSO, 1984.

Donzelot, J. *The Policing of Families*, Hutchinson, 1979.

Douglas, M. *In the Active Voice*, RKP, 1982.

Douglas, M. (ed.) *Food in the Social Order*, Russell Sage Foundation, 1984.

Doyal, L. *The Political Economy of Health*, Pluto, 1981.

Fisher, M.F.K. *The Art of Eating*, Picador, 1983.
Goody, J. *Cooking, Cuisine and Class*, Cambridge University Press, 1982.
Hayter, T. *The Creation of World Poverty*, Pluto, 1981.
Kerr, M. and Charles, N. 'Servers and providers: the distribution of food within the family', in *Sociological Review*, vol. 34, no. 1, 1986.
Lawrence, M. *The Anorexic Experience*, Women's Press, 1984.
Lévi-Strauss, C. 'The culinary triangle', in *New Society*, December 1966, pp. 937–940.
Mack, J. and Lansley, S. *Poor Britain*, George Allen and Unwin, 1985.
MacLeod, S. *The Art of Starvation*, Virago, 1981.
McIntosh, M. 'The family, regulation and the public sphere', in *State and Society in Contemporary Britain*, G. McLennan *et al.* (eds), Polity Press, 1984.
Ministry of Agriculture, Fisheries and Food *Household Food Consumption and Expenditure: 1982*, HMSO, 1984.
Murcott, A. 'On the social significance of the "cooked dinner" in South Wales', in *Social Science Information*, vol. 21, no. 4/5, 1982.
Murcott, A. 'Cooking and the cooked: a note on the domestic preparation of meals', in *The Sociology of Food and Eating*, A. Murcott (ed.), Gower, 1983.
NACNE (National Advisory Committee on Nutrition Education) *Proposals for Nutritional Guidelines for Health Education in Britain*, Health Education Council, 1983.
Newson, J. and E. *Four Years Old in an Urban Community*, Penguin, 1970.
Newson, J. and E. *Seven Years Old in the Home Environment*, George Allen and Unwin, 1976.
NFS (see Ministry of Agriculture, Fisheries and Food).
Nicod, M. 'Gastronomically speaking: food studied as a medium of communication', in *Nutrition and Lifestyles*, M. Turner (ed), Applied Science Publishers, 1980.
Oakley, A. *Sex, Gender and Society*, Temple Smith, 1982.
Orbach, S. *Fat is a Feminist Issue*, Hamlyn Paperbacks, 1981.
Pember-Reeves, M. *Round about a Pound a Week*, Virago, 1984.
Rowntree, S. *How the Labourer Lives*, Nelson, 1913.
Sharpe, S. *'Just Like a Girl' How Girls Learn to be Women*, Penguin, 1978.
Shostak, M. *Nisa*, Penguin, 1983.
Spender, D. *Man Made Language*, RKP, 1985.
Spring Rice, M. *Working-class Wives*, Virago, 1981.
Tudge, C. *The Famine Business*, Pelican, 1979.
Twigg, J. 'Vegetarianism and the meanings of meat', in *The Sociology of Food and Eating*, A. Murcott (ed.), Gower, 1983.
Wardle, C. *Changing Food Habits in the UK*, 1977.
Wilson, E. *Women and the Welfare State*, Tavistock, 1977.
Wright, H. *Swallow it Whole*, New Statesman Report No. 4, 1981.

Index